TICKET TO MADLAND

How I Went Insane and Met New People

A MEMOIR BY

JOCELYN DAVIS

Beringer Books

ISBN 979-8-9914459-0-0 (paperback)
ISBN 979-8-9914459-1-7 (ebook)

Beringer Books

Publisher's Cataloging-in-Publication Data

Names: Davis, Jocelyn, author.
Title: Ticket to madland : how I went insane and met new people /
Jocelyn Davis.
Description: Santa Fe, NM: Beringer Books, 2024.
Identifiers: LCCN: 2024918190 | ISBN: 979-8-9914459-0-0 (paper-
back) | 979-8-9914459-1-7 (ebook)
Subjects: LCSH Davis, Jocelyn. | Davis, Jocelyn--Mental health. |
Mentally ill--United States--Biography. | BISAC BIOGRAPHY
& AUTOBIOGRAPHY / Memoirs | BIOGRAPHY &
AUTOBIOGRAPHY / Medical
Classification: LCC RC464 .D38 2024 | DDC 616.8900/92--dc23

"Alice" quotations are from Lewis Carroll's *Alice in Wonderland* and
Through the Looking Glass (public domain).

Author's Disclaimer: This book is an account of my own experiences
as I remember them. It is not meant to be used, nor should it be used,
as a substitute for medical advice or to diagnose or treat any medical
or psychological condition.

PRAISE FOR *TICKET TO MADLAND*

Ticket to Madland reads like a medical thriller. Jocelyn Davis perfectly captures what happens when the most ancient part of your brain, sensing physical weakness, suddenly rears up to pull you through the looking glass into a distorted, nightmarish, funhouse world. It's a page-turning, wryly observed, beautifully written chronicle of how the most put-together of us is vulnerable to being tipped over when there's a perfect storm, and what we learn on the way back.

—**Deborah Grace Winer,** theater artist; author of *The Night and the Music* and *On the Sunny Side of the Street*

Davis says she wrote the book in order to "demystify, destigmatize, and defang" the experience of mental illness, creating a "small, clear window" in the wall surrounding Madland. She succeeds, brilliantly. You'll be informed, entertained, and inspired by this true story of a mental healing journey.

—**Tal Leead, PsyD,** psychologist; author of *Happier Being: Your Path to Optimizing Habits, Health & Happiness*

Ticket to Madland is a powerful memoir that blends vivid storytelling with refreshing humor. As a mental health expert with a background in neuroscience, I highly recommend this book for its authentic and touching portrayal of mental health struggles. Davis's compassionate and insightful perspective offers a deeper understanding of psychiatric illness and the resilience it takes to find hope amid chaos. Her story is a testament to the human spirit and the power of humor in adversity. A must-read.

—**Srini Pillay, MD,** psychiatrist and CEO, NeuroBusiness Group; author of *Tinker Dabble Doodle Try: Unlock the Power of the Unfocused Mind*

ALSO BY JOCELYN DAVIS

For Matt, who made me tea.

For Emily, who sent me lion-face emojis.

And for Sylvia, who sat by the rabbit hole and called my name.

"But I don't want to go among mad people," Alice remarked.

"Oh, you can't help that," said the Cat; "we're all mad here."

—Lewis Carroll, *Alice in Wonderland*

"A slow sort of country!" said the Queen. "Now, *here,* you see, it takes all the running you can do to keep in the same place. If you want to get somewhere else, you must run at least twice as fast as that!"

—Lewis Carroll, *Through the Looking Glass*

"It's a fabulous monster!" the Unicorn cried out, before Alice could reply.

"Then hand round the plum cake, Monster," the Lion said.

—*Through the Looking Glass*

CONTENTS

PART III: DOWN THE RABBIT HOLE

PART IV: THE DOOR IN THE WALL

THE MONSTERS OF MADLAND

Mental illness is another country. Like all countries it is populated, but in it you don't meet people so much as encounter them: monsters in a fairy-tale forest.

"How curious," you think as the monsters approach, noses snuffling, heads atilt. Some are belligerent, others calm. Some stare, others look away. Some have crisp white coats, stethoscopes, and an air of detachment; others have frazzled hair and a tendency to howl. While most keep a few paces distant, a few come close enough for you to touch—were it permitted. There are a lot of rules in Madland. "No touching" is one of the biggest.

Madland is separated from Saneland by a looking glass. At first the glass is permeable, gauzy, allowing you to go back and forth many times a day, but as time passes it thickens like gelatin, then like glue. Your own monstrous face confronts you as you push on the glass trying to return. Failing. Soon you start to wonder whether Saneland ever existed. You get used to the hopelessness, the way you can't seem to walk in your intended direction no matter how resolutely you set off, so you decide it's best simply to walk in circles or, finally, to drop to the ground and never move again. What's the use, you think. There's no way out.

I first glimpsed Madland in January 2018, entered it for real in July 2020, and left it (maybe permanently, maybe not) fifteen weeks after that. Up till that time I had been, to quote the words a doctor once wrote on my chart, "alert, cooperative,

1

well-groomed." A top-grade student with two master's degrees. A successful business executive turned book author. A reliable woman with a loving family, kind friends, and ample resources. Sure, a couple of minor medical problems, bit of an anxious personality, occasionally prone to panic attacks, but overall in great shape, my act solidly together.

Then, at age 57 and with barely a warning, I found myself on a steam train to hell. The final weeks of that bouncing, shrieking, sleepless journey were crammed horizon to horizon with horror, stuffed wall to wall with suffering, filled hour by interminable hour with grinding, nauseating fear. I was insane. I was suicidal. It was excruciating.

"What caused this collapse?" you ask. "An infection? Genetic condition? Brain tumor?"

No, no, and no.

"Trauma, then. Something dreadful must have happened to you."

Nope. This is not a trauma memoir, and although I did eventually receive a diagnosis for one of my more overt symptoms, the reasons for the psychiatric nosedive remain less than clear. When I asked the neurologist at the Mayo Clinic for a theory, he waved a hand and said, "You just got in a funk." Well … having experienced the funk, I can offer a more complete account than that; nevertheless, all I can say with certainty about my trip to Madland is, I went.

I believe it's the same for many, perhaps most, mental illnesses. One minute you're riding your usual commuter train, preparing to get off at your usual stop, the weather fine, a pleasant evening planned; the next minute you're disembarking onto a rain-slick platform in a strange city at night, your bags gone missing, your heart pounding, your cold clammy fingers clutching a ticket you don't remember having bought. You've arrived in the Bad Place, the Unhappiest Place on Earth. Why? Who knows. How to get home becomes your all-consuming concern, but there is no map, no schedule, and no trains seem to be leaving. Worst of all, the people (monsters?) swarming past you in the station act as if there's nothing wrong: they smile and offer to take your picture, tell you you're looking well, and when you go to the traveler's aid booth the friendly man-monster behind the glass indicates a QR code you can scan to find the local attractions. When you start to cry, he sighs and shoves a grubby sheaf of forms at you.

"What's this?" you ask, sniffling.

"A contract," he says, "promising you won't throw yourself onto the tracks. It's illegal in these parts, you know. Sign here, and here."

It's a bewildering, scary mess of a country, perhaps especially to those who haven't been. Which brings me to this book's three purposes: to demystify, destigmatize, and defang.

First, I want to **demystify** the processes of mental illness and recovery.* Western popular culture likes to tell tales of cruel villains or crushing diseases that induce violent psychosis in their victims. Movies such as *Sybil, The Shining, A Beautiful Mind,* and *One Flew over the Cuckoo's Nest* shape our view of insanity's causes, demeanor, and treatment; the words "mental patient" summon to mind Jack Nicholson reeling down a hotel hallway with an axe, Russell Crowe strapped writhing to a gurney. Most

---

* A terminology note: *Behavioral health* is today's term for what used to be called mental or psychiatric health. I don't like it. I was not made ill by misbehavior, and although some of the people I met had self-medicated with alcohol or other drugs, that behavior was not the cause of their illness but the result. Moreover, *behavioral health* serves to perpetuate the old, pernicious idea that nutcases could solve their problems if only they'd stop making poor choices. *Neurodivergence* is another fashionable term I dislike, because it suggests that devastating sicknesses are really just fun quirks of personality that acceptance can transform into non-issues. I will therefore be using *mental illness, brain disease, psychiatric disorder,* even *insanity*—words that most actual psych patients seem to prefer.

psychiatric patients and situations, of course, aren't anything like that. Yes, trauma-induced dysfunction is a grim reality for many; abusive authority figures abound; psychotic episodes are a thing. Such stories are told and should be told. What we get less often, though, are stories of quieter madness caused by, what? A chemical imbalance, a frayed neural net, hormone fluctuations, a lurking virus—or nothing discernable.

A friend's elderly mother, in excellent shape for her age, suddenly went (to use her word for it) "cuckoo." Doctors tested her for stroke, heart problems, infection, cancer, you name it, but found nothing. She spent three months in a state of abject confusion, non-communicative, with no idea where she was or what was happening. Then she made a complete recovery. The doctors still can't explain it; her daughter suspects low sodium was the culprit.

When I look back at my time in Madland, I do see some reeling and writhing, some violently damaged souls and a few coldly calloused ones; mostly, though, I see a lot of caring, competent medical pros going to work every day and trying their best, within the limits of a flawed system, to treat a lot of perfectly ordinary, unaccountably screwed-up patients who persist bravely in seeking treatment for their ill-understood conditions. I see a world where heads are lost and restored as a matter of routine. A world of pain, yes, and many mysteries, but a world, too, of kindness, diligence, and reason.

Second, I want to help **destigmatize** mental illness. Greater understanding of substance abuse allows many of us to say, "I'm an alcoholic" or "addict" without fear of judgment, but few of us are as accepting or open when it comes to the diseases that can underlie substance abuse: depression, anxiety, obsessive compulsive disorder, ADHD, schizoaffective disorder, bipolar disorder, etcetera. The shame associated with revealing an "abnormality" can be intense, so people who suffer from such problems tend to keep mum about them. And while some of us with brains gone wild manage to hunt down a diagnosis, many of us are told our sickness is "idiopathic": medical shorthand for "Dunno why you're like this but try these drugs."

A friend I'll call Toni* has struggled for most of her life with generalized anxiety and panic disorder—idiopathic, as that disorder usually is. You wouldn't know it if you met her casually: she comes across as smart, accomplished, and bubbly. She told me about the time she confessed to her therapist her desire to date, along with her fear it was out of the question. The therapist suggested she go on a dating site and, upon meeting someone, tell him about her condition.

"Yeah, right," said Toni. "Like I'd ever do that."

"Well, what's the worst that could happen?" said the therapist. "I'm not saying you have to do it. Just think about it."

Toni thought about it and decided to give the impossible a try. She found a nice-seeming guy online and met him for lunch. After a minute or two of small talk she took a deep breath and said, "I want to be open with you about something. I suffer from an anxiety disorder."

"Oh, me too," said the guy, chewing a breadstick. "How do you cope with yours?"

They spent the rest of lunch comparing notes.

Like Toni, I come across as smart, accomplished, and—OK, not bubbly, let's just say *amiable*. Yet my own anxiety problem, worsened by several others, took me on a journey that wove through a dozen doctors' offices to a rehab center and finally to a hospital, where I stayed for two weeks locked up with other psychiatric patients. I used to pity those people. Now, I see them as my people. *Ich bin ein Madlander.*

Third and last, I want to **defang** the "prowde spirits" who, according to Sir Thomas More, "cannot bear to be mocked." I

---

* Except for my immediate family members, all names of individuals and institutions have been changed.

didn't used to believe in spirits and am not sure I do now, but just as there are no atheists in foxholes, there are no atheists in a psych ward. Neither I nor any of my hospitalized comrades scoffed at the woman with bipolarism and no teeth, who described in vivid detail the hour when a demon had taken possession of her home, then her body. She insisted only Jesus could cure her. Maybe she was right. They say hell is separation from God, and there were hours, days, when I was convinced I'd been cut off from divine grace, that the entire world consisted solely of me, Unbearable Me, cowering 24/7 under a blazing orange eye.

There is no self-propelled escape from the prison of the self, so I'm pretty sure some type of benevolent supernatural intervention, whether of god or goddess, angels or saints or ancestors, aided medical skill in getting me out of that prison. Moreover, I'm open to the idea that malevolent supernatural forces abetted scrambled neurons in putting me there in the first place. Such malevolent forces want more than anything to be taken seriously, dead seriously, as they scream, "Off with her head!"—so I intend to mock the crap out of them, and if this comes across as laughing at the sick and their caregivers, so be it. Not only do funny things happen both in and on the way to psych wards, but a sense of humor, it turns out, is a strength of many mental patients; during my sojourn we laughed at one another, at ourselves, and most of all at the prowde spirits, who were not amused. I trust you will be.

Demystify, destigmatize, defang. I don't imagine this book will tear down the wall of misgivings and misunderstanding that surrounds the monsters of Madland, but it may make a small clear window in that wall, which will be enough.

PART I

Off
with Her
Head

CHAPTER 1

THE WALRUS AND
THE CARPENTER

What the—Jesus, zip up your pants!

Having exited the bathroom and handed off my urine sample to the ER nurse, I glanced down to see the panty part of my pantyhose showing through a wide-open fly. Earlier that afternoon, before leaving for the hospital, I'd put on the tan tights under my jeans in the vague expectation that the psych ward authorities would let me keep them on after admission, thus facilitating my plan to have the means handy in case I decided, finally and truly, to kill myself. (Plus it was a chilly November and I believe in layering.) So nothing was really exposed; still, the gaping fly made Sane Me wince. It was Sane Me who had barked out the zip-pants order.

Sane Me had been issuing directives to Mad Me for the past three months, give or take a week, and working together we had managed to sustain a performance of alert, cooperative, well-groomed normality. But at sunrise that morning I'd stuffed myself into my big coat to set out for a walk, the first of the day's seven or eight, and made it most of the way across the kitchen before crumpling in a heap on the floor at the top of the basement stairs. I hadn't lost my balance. The last dregs of my willpower were gone.

My husband, Matt, came up the stairs a minute later and found me like that. "What're you doing, Bear?" he asked.

"Hospital, hospital, hospital," I whispered.

There ensued a muddled stretch of time in which Matt persuaded me to wait until he could talk to my psychiatrist, we waited till her office opened at eight, he called and was informed that Dr. Funar couldn't talk to him unless I gave my written permission, we drove all the way down Cerrillos Road to the clinic so I could sign away my privacy rights, then drove back home and waited some more. When Dr. Funar phoned, Matt spoke with her. She agreed the situation sounded unmanageable and confirmed that St. Giles had a bed in their psych ward. Matt told me to get ready to go. I packed a bag with a hodgepodge of mostly inappropriate items: spiral-bound crossword puzzle books, electronic devices, bottles of pills, drawstring pajamas, an extra pair of tights, and my stuffed elephant (name: Elephant). We drove to the hospital, registered, and waited for a long time in the grim chairs of the outer ER. I watched a couple who were having a baby check in at the desk; the woman was wearing a magenta bathrobe and pink fuzzy slippers. Matt patted my knee as I fiddled with the white plastic barcode bracelet they'd snapped onto my left wrist. We were called into triage, asked questions ("How often do you have thoughts of suicide: never, hardly ever, sometimes, often, every day?"), dismissed to wait again, and finally ushered back to the main zone, where after another very long wait I described my plight to a bespectacled nurse who brought me a Saran-wrapped ham sandwich on white bread with mustard then placed us in a holding room with a black-padded bed and an orange plastic chair. My blood was drawn for the Covid test, my urine accepted for the drug test.

Now I had reseated myself on the bed, fly zipped, Elephant clutched to my chest, the crusts of the sandwich beside me. Matt was sitting on the orange chair reading Gibbon's *Decline and Fall of the Roman Empire* on my Kindle. I was feeling wanly hopeful that somewhere in the building was a solution to … everything. The ground wasn't bouncing (much); my scalp wasn't itching (much); and thanks to Sane Me's firm hold on the reins, I was able to keep still (sort of). It was three p.m. on November 4, 2020, the day after Election Day.

The glass-fronted holding rooms around the ER's perimeter seemed mostly unoccupied: strange, I thought, given that the pandemic was peaking here in Santa Fe. People in blue or pink scrubs walked around the gym-sized oval and leaned over desks in the central corral, quietly doing things. A couple of paramedics rolled in a gurney with an elderly woman on it; they spoke sotto voce to a doctor, who rolled the gurney away. Nobody was rushing about yelling "Stat!"—not like on TV, I thought, pinching the nose wire of my facemask. The place looked clean enough but smelled like a gas station convenience store, probably due to the ham sandwich and the bathroom across from me, its door open, its floor littered with paper towels.

To my right was an inner room with a lockable door, also open, and in that room, lying on a high bed like mine, was a man. All I could see of him were his calves and boots: work boots of stiff ochre leather with thick beige tread and round toes. Though the rest of his body was hidden from view, I knew he was large, because of his large boots, and passed-out drunk, because of his stertorous snores. I imagined he might work in construction: a carpenter of some sort, good with tools. I did not want him to wake up, but in another forty minutes or so—we were still waiting for the results of my Covid test—he did wake up and shambled forth, looking like a Yeti or some similarly huge shaggy creature, reeking of alcohol, maskless. Taking no notice of us, he gripped the jamb of the holding-room doorway and bellowed:

"Hey! HEYYY! I wanna go home!"

Immediately a couple of nurses hurried over and guided him back to his bed. A security guard wasn't far behind. I listened, apprehensive, to the voices coming from the inner room.

"OK, big guy, you're OK. You need to stay here, OK?"

"I need a shot! I need it! The anxiety, it's so bad ... oh my god ..."

"We know, we know. We're going to get you your shot, hon. Just a few more minutes."

The Carpenter's tone grew desperate. "Please, I just wanna go home! *Please!*"

"We have to check you out first, hon. Sit down, OK? You need to stay here. Try to relax. Breathe with me, now. Slow, deep breaths."

"Oh God—oh God—it's like I'm going crazy! Please, please, gimme my shot!"

"We're gonna get you your shot. You're OK, big guy."

The voices of the nurses and security guard were unperturbed, even cheerful. It was obvious the Carpenter could lay them out with a punch and make a run for it should he choose, but equally obvious he would not do that because they were in complete control. They made no move to restrain him or to lock the door, which I appreciated; I did not want any doors locked on me, either, though I knew it was going to happen eventually. Psych wards are locked wards.

Soon a nurse emerged and asked if we'd mind moving out into the hallway. "It's just that we have a bit of a situation here," she said. Of course, we said, and gathered my things. As we settled ourselves again on orange plastic chairs, along came another man: pale skinned, fat bellied, with bulbous eyes and unkempt gray hair, clothed in a rumpled work shirt, sweatpants, and backless slippers. I'd seen this man strolling around earlier and had assumed he was a fellow patient, possibly a homeless person awaiting admission. Now, though, it became clear that this walrus-like individual was a hospital employee. Trailed by a tall, fit-looking woman with short spiky blonde hair, he passed through the holding room to the inner room and began to speak to the Carpenter:

"Hey there, I'm [inaudible], the crisis counselor here. How's it going?"

"I wanna leave! I want my shot!"

"Sure, we'll get you your shot," said the Walrus. "Can you tell me how you're feeling?"

"Bad! Ohhh God! I'm, I'm … it's like I'm going crazy!"

"I understand. We're here to help you."

The Carpenter continued to rant. I stopped listening and turned to Matt. "That's me," I said.

"What? Who's you?"

"That drunk guy in there. I'm him."

Matt looked skeptical. "You're nothing like him, Woolly." (Woolly Bear is my pet name, deriving from an occasion decades ago when I'd remarked on the woolly-bear caterpillar's ability to predict winter temperatures with the thickness of its red band, a fact well known to readers of Laura Ingalls Wilder but that had struck Matt as hilariously obscure.)

"We're the same," I insisted. "That's how I feel on the inside. But on the outside I'm this nice polite woman, and he's a big loud scary man."

"That's not the only difference," said Matt.

"Still. I'm him." I hugged Elephant tighter, frowning, thinking about being alert, cooperative, and well-groomed, thinking about the times in the past couple weeks when I'd howled, just like the Carpenter, with no abatement of terror. *Just sit, sweetie,* said Sane Me, *just sit.**

---

* Sane Me wasn't an actual voice in my head. She was more like an energy: a vibration of reason, experience, and wry humor, which, thank goodness, abandoned me only a few times in the whole journey.

The Walrus emerged, slippers flapping, followed by his tall blonde henchwoman and a nurse. The three stood a few yards away from us, conferring.

"I thought that guy was a patient," Matt whispered.

"So did I," I whispered back. "But he's not. He's the crisis counselor."

Walrus, Blonde Henchwoman, and Nurse walked away. I don't know what happened to the Carpenter after that; maybe he got his shot (he stopped yelling), but I didn't have time to wonder because another nurse approached and said my Covid test was negative so we could go on back now to the Behavioral Health intake area. As we followed her down a hallway, I felt a nudge in the ribs from Sane Me: *Show the nice nurse you've got it together.*

"What's your name?" I asked, smiling.

"I'm Joanna," she said, turning her head and smiling back.

"Hi, Joanna, I'm Jocelyn. It's nice to meet you."

"Nice to meet you, too."

I maintained good posture as we walked deeper into the hospital maze.

———

Nurse Joanna wasn't smiling anymore. I kept one hand on my purse, the other on my backpack, as she stood over me and Matt in the cramped intake office, explaining again that I would have to give up all my stuff to be inventoried and the time for me to give it all up was right now.

"Yes, but, I only brought what's *allowed*," I said, trying to keep my voice steady. I had been in a healing center (trendy name for a rehab facility) only three weeks before and thought I knew the drill: no alcohol, no drugs, no tech devices, nothing sharp. Except for my prescriptions—well, plus my phone and Kindle—I hadn't brought anything like that.

"They're pretty much only going to let you keep your clothes," said Joanna, stone-faced.

"But I need, like, my glasses and my contact lenses and my wallet and my toothbrush. I *need* them."

"Anything that's allowed will be given back to you. But I have to take it all now. You should give your wallet and any valuables, like jewelry, to your husband to take home."

"Um, OK, yes ..." *Cooperative!* I began to fumble with my rings, then stopped, bent over, and fished out of my backpack the medium plastic baggie containing my glasses and contact lens paraphernalia, plus the large plastic baggie containing my many prescription pill bottles. I took my wallet from my purse. I piled baggies and wallet on top of Elephant in my lap. "Maybe I should separate out the stuff I need to keep? I brought extra plastic bags." I cast a desperate glance at Matt, seated next to me.

Nurse Joanna shook her head. "All medications must come from our pharmacy."

"I see, but ..." *Do not freak out.*

"Is there another way to go about this?" asked Matt. "I think she'd like to keep her stuff for now, if that's all right."

Abruptly, unaccountably, Joanna shifted tack. "Yes," she said, looking at Matt and smiling. "I'll take the meds and she can hang onto the rest and give it straight to the nurses in the ward once she's down there. They'll do the inventory."

"That sounds good," Matt said. "Thank you."

"Yes!" I said. "I'd rather do that. Thank you!"

"Fine." Stoneface again. "The nurse will be right in to do your intake." She went to the door, swiped her ID card through a chrome box above the handle, and exited.

A whoosh of relief drowned out a mouse-squeak of fear. (Why did she have to swipe her card to get out of the room?) *Never mind. You can keep your stuff for now.* (But why?)

A few minutes later, the intake nurse arrived. Making no introduction, she sat down at the desk, pulled up a file on her computer, and began to recite my medications. I wondered where the information, which was at least a month out of date, had come from. Nurse No-name kept shaking her head, lips thin, as I corrected her: "No, I'm not taking Lexapro; I take Zoloft, 25 milligrams, that was Dr. Funar. No mirtazapine. No nortriptyline. I'm taking Ambien CR, 12.5 milligrams, right, the bigger dose, that's what Dr. Funar prescribed me for sleep. And acyclovir, it's an antiviral, 200 milligrams five times a day. Yes, *five* times a day, that's prescribed by my ENT, Dr. Greene ... Why? He thinks I have herpes zoster and that's what causes the vertigo. No, I'm not doing the quetiapine; I was on it for a few days, but I stopped. Hydroxyzine, yes, that's Dr. Ortega, three times a day as needed. And the hormones: estradiol patch, point-one milligram—no, not point oh five, that's out of date, now it's point one—plus 100 milligrams progesterone, no, not norethindrone, I switched back to progesterone a couple months ago ... Yes, that's right ... Yes, I'm sure." *Babe, we may be insane, but we know our meds.*

Nurse No-name typed fast, squinting at the screen. Once she had the drugs down, she confirmed my doctors: Ortega, primary care; Greene, ENT; Funar, psychiatrist.

"Dr. Andersen?"

"He's a neurologist; I only saw him once." (Cuz I didn't like him cuz he yelled at me to stop looking at my notes and he said I have vestibular migraine which I don't)

More fast typing. Her phone beeped; she glanced at it then looked directly at me for the first time and said, "I'm sorry, I just have to take care of something real quick. Be right back." She rose and left the room, swiping her card through the chrome box above the door handle.

After the door swung shut, I sat staring at the chrome box.

I got up, went to the door, and pushed down hard on the handle. It did not give.

Trembling, I turned to Matt. "The door is locked from the *inside!* It's *locked!*"

Matt nodded, once. "Of course it's locked. We're in the mental health area now."

I walked back to my chair, sat down, stood up, sat down. "I don't think I can do this. I don't want to be in here." I felt the dreadful electric tidewaters starting to flood my body.

"It's a room like any other room." Exasperation tightened his voice.

A room like any other room. A room like any other room. He's right. What are you going to do? Pound on the door, tell them you're leaving? At this point they probably won't let you leave. Anyway, you know Matt can't take this anymore. You can't go home. Jesus Christ, girl, get a grip.

I drew a deep breath, let it out. I looked around the office: Floor. Ceiling. Walls. Window. Desk. Chairs. Computer. "It's a room like any other room."

"Yes," said Matt.

Listen to me. You need to be here. You chose to come here. You are choosing this.

I slumped and dropped my head, miming surrender. If I didn't look at the door, or the lock box, didn't look at them or think about them, maybe it'd be all right.

The door swung open and Nurse No-name reentered, sat, typed a few more things into the computer, then faced us: "So, the next step is to take you into a pre-entry room. They're not quite ready for you in the ward, it'll be about 45 minutes."

"What kind of room is it? Is it locked? Can he" (a glance at Matt) "come with me?"

"It's just a small waiting room. Yes, it's locked. No, he can't come. It won't be for that long, though."

"I don't want to be in a locked room. I don't … no …" I was starting to sound like the Carpenter. A sudden, terrible thought hit me. "Are the bedrooms in the *ward* locked?"

"Oh no, no, the bedrooms aren't locked. The ward is very spacious." Her voice grew cheery. "There's a big sunny dayroom with a big window that looks out over the mountains. It's a great view. Some of our patients just sit and look out the window all day!"

Into my head popped an image of gowned, drooling zombies staring at mountain scenery. Nurse No-name eyed me as I sat with twisting hands, my breath coming faster. She said, "Wait just a minute, I'll be right back" and left the room again.

I waited. *You're choosing this. You're choosing this. It's a room like any other room. Floor, ceiling, walls, window, desk, chairs, computer, door, door—*

The door reopened and No-Name reappeared, followed by …

The Walrus! And his Blonde Henchwoman! Slippers a-flap, he shuffled over and seated himself at the desk with an "oof" while Henchwoman took up a stance against the far wall with hands behind her back, posture military, expression severe. Sane Me (who is not only bossy and judgmental, but also easily amused) started to chuckle: *Lord have mercy, it's the crisis counselor! He's here to talk you off the ledge. And his blonde goon is here to tackle you if you make a run for it. Back off, blonde goon!*

The Walrus's pale eyes goggled at me over his facemask. He spoke pleasantly, calmly, just as he had to the Carpenter: "Hello, Jocelyn, I'm [mumble-mumble], the hospital crisis counselor. You want to tell me what's going on?"

The time has come, the Walrus said, to talk of many things: of shoes, and ships, and sealing wax … I sat up straight and began to pour out my woes: the vertigo, the insomnia, the constant torturous anxiety, the patches of nerve pain, the unbearable itching, the noises driving through my head like knives, the predawn terror, the thoughts of suicide. The Walrus remained silent, making notes on his yellow pad as I burbled on: "… and so I haven't really slept in three months, and, I don't know, I've tried everything, nothing works, but I don't want to be locked in, and I just, I just, I just need *help,*" I concluded, helplessly.

"OK, we're going to get you help," said the Walrus in his best reassure-the-maniac tone. He made a few more notes on his yellow pad. "How about if you and your husband go from here to another waiting area? You won't be locked in. You'll need to sit in a holding room, like the one you were in before, until they're ready to admit you. Does that work?"

"Oh … yes. Thank you. That works." I rubbed my thighs in long, nervous strokes.

Yes, that works, said Sane Me with a judicious nod. *Well done, Walrus.* (Sane Me is tough but fair. She recognizes competence.)

"And I can go with her?" asked Matt.

"You can. But when they take her down to the ward, that'll be it; you can't go there."

"I understand," said Matt. "Thank you."

"No problem." The Walrus heaved himself to his feet, conferred briefly with Nurse No-name, and exited the room, slippers flapping, Blonde Henchwoman trailing close behind.

The new waiting area was a short hallway with a staff office and TV alcove on the left, three patient rooms on the right. As in Dante's Limbo, the air was dim and still.

Nurse No-name accompanied us there; she left the sliding glass door to the holding room open but said we had to stay inside. I asked if I could go to the bathroom and, having received permission, took my eye paraphernalia in their baggie, went down the hall, leaned over the sink, plucked out my contacts, put them in their case, and put on my glasses. I wasn't sure, but I was starting to see that a psych ward was several jumps past a rehab center and suspecting that now might be the last time in a long time I'd have access to a mirror. On returning from the bathroom, I saw a man in the TV alcove hunched on a couch with a blanket draped over his shoulders. A cut on his head was oozing blood. As I passed, he shouted something at the TV. Was he one of the men currently in the ward? "We have three gentlemen and two ladies," Nurse No-name had said. I wondered if the Carpenter would be there, too.

Our new holding room was tiny, with just enough space for a bed and, oddly, a massive reclining chair. I perched on the bed, and Matt stood next to me, looking worried. Well, of course he was worried, he'd been worried for a solid three months, but was he afraid that coming here had been a mistake? In recent weeks, Drs. Ortega and Funar had both advised me *not* to go to the hospital. Dr. Ortega said, *They'll just put you in with a bunch of Covid patients.* Dr. Funar said, *They'll just load you up on medications and release you.* True, Dr. Funar had changed her mind that morning and said I should go, but that was only because things had seemed so dire. Matt knew mornings were my worst time; no doubt he was thinking he'd overreacted to my dawn collapse and now here he was, about to stash his wife in the loony bin. Thanks to his years as a college dean dealing with students who needed crisis care, he was of the opinion that St. Giles did nothing more than keep struggling people for a day or two then "kick them out on the street." He wasn't a big fan of the place.

He stood with arms crossed, head down, under the school clock stuck high on the wall. I reached out and patted his shoulder. "Don't worry," I said. "This is the right thing to do."

"I hope so." He did not sound optimistic.

Since July sixteenth, when the mal debarquement vertigo had struck again and I'd found myself back in Boat World—the ground bouncing, swaying, tilting under me as in a moderate ocean chop, never stopping, worse when I sat still, worst of all when I lay down and closed my eyes—Matt had been an anchor in the storm: steady, patient, and empathetic. In childhood he'd had to cope with an unstable mother and father (the film *Who's Afraid of Virginia Woolf* was cathartic for him, he said, because it reminded him so much of his parents), which experience, along with his stints as dean, had given him plenty of practice managing volatile types. As summer passed and I stopped sleeping,

20

began spiraling, and grew more and more frantic, he remained calm. Ceding the bedroom to me, he slept in the basement office and, "Just come downstairs and find me if you're scared," he'd say, "wake me up, I don't mind." A few weeks ago he'd taken over dinner duty, bringing a plate to me each evening as I sat in the battered armchair in our daughter's old room, staring at Netflix shows with dwindling comprehension. He made me mug after mug of tea: mint, ginger, licorice, chamomile. And he stuck to his opinion that I was not crazy; he'd seen plenty of crazy people, he said, and I wasn't like them, I was just "having difficulties."

But. There were those three times he had lost it. The first had been in late September, when I'd returned from a walk during which I'd called the national suicide hotline and spoken with a sympathetic woman who, after listening to me babble and wail for nearly an hour, inquired whether I had "a plan." When I told her hanging myself with a scarf seemed like the way to go (literally), she suggested I put all my scarves in a box, tape it up, and place it somewhere inaccessible. Sane Me thought this a pretty dumb idea; still, she could see the point, and it was a step to take—Sane Me was constantly looking for steps to take—so once I got home, I tiptoed around gathering up my scarves of all varieties, found a cardboard box, and dumped the lot on the kitchen counter. I was just trying to remember where the duct tape was when I heard Matt's step behind me. I froze.

"What's all this, Bear?" His tone was light, faintly amused.

Sound rational! "Uh, well, I called the sui ... the crisis hotline ... on my walk ... and the person said it might help if, if I took all my, all my scarves and put them in a box and tape it up and, um, hide it somewhere so that, you know, they'll be harder for me to get at ... um ..."

I trailed off. I could see his head exploding in slow motion. *Uh-oh, here we go.*

"All right that's IT!" His hands flung out, chopping at the air; his eyes bulged, his voice ascended an octave. "This has to stop!

21

Do you hear me?! That is *enough*! This whole thing has got to stop *right now*! This whole ridiculous thing! You need to SNAP OUT OF IT!"

> **Mad Me:** Oh my god oh my god please stop yelling please stop yelling

> **Sane Me:** *Ha! I knew he'd say "snap out of it" eventually. Just like Cher in* Moonstruck. *A lot of people love that movie. Me, I never cared for it.*

His tirade continued for another thirty seconds or so. I circled him slowly, maintaining eye contact as one might with a snarling dog. I kept saying, "Yes. OK. Yes." I reached the sink, stopped there, leaned on the white stone rim, and looked out the window at the adobe stucco wall of the neighbors' house. Up down, up down, up down went the floor.

His demeanor calmed. He came and stood beside me. "I mean, I really think you have to pull yourself together. Don't you think? You can't keep doing this, Woolly. You need to try and snap out of it. Right? Don't you think?"

"Yes," I said. I turned my head to look at him. Silence filled the space between us. I was thinking: You have no idea of the impossibility of what you're asking.

Suddenly he laughed. "You look just like Sebastian."

"I do? Really?" It was a high compliment: Sebastian, the hopeless alcoholic aristocrat in *Brideshead Revisited,* is played in the miniseries by the gorgeous Anthony Andrews.

"Yes. He's so handsome, and you're so beautiful. You look just like him right now."

"Ha, like when Charles says, I'm no help, am I? and Sebastian says, No, no help."

"Exactly."

We both smiled. He said to give him the scarves, he'd take charge of them. He placed the bundle—I learned much later—on a shelf in his closet in plain sight. I didn't hunt for them; after all, I still had tights, shawls, a dog leash, belts, phone cords ... oh, one finds all sorts of ropey things lying around a house when one starts to look.

He had two more meltdowns after that: one in late October that featured the statement, "I don't give a *flying fuck* if you don't want to take the drugs!" and another on November third, just yesterday, that had him screaming, "I *hate* you for doing this to me!" as I lay supine in bed in a black dawn, drenched with flop sweat, sick with terror. I did not blame him; not then, not today. Rather, I recognized fits of panic not unlike my own. He was being pushed to the brink.

Now, as I looked at him standing under the wall clock in the hospital holding room, I heard Sane Me say again: *He can't take this anymore. You cannot go home. You must stay here.*

The clock hands were pointing to twelve and six when an orderly showed up with two trays. "Dinner! Where would you like it?" Having had nothing to eat since the ham sandwich, I was glad someone had thought to send us a meal. The orderly set the trays down on the bed with hearty good cheer: "Salisbury steak, my favorite!" We thanked him. He left.

I eased myself into the recliner, tray on lap, eyeing the mangled oval of meat with slimy slosh of brown gravy. On the side were boiled carrots, mashed potatoes, and a bowl of limp lettuce with a packet of Italian dressing. Apple juice and water to drink. Oatmeal raisin cookie for dessert. Is there anyone on earth who actually likes oatmeal raisin cookies? *Too bad!* Sane Me snarled. *Eat it, eat it all. What did you expect, your mother's cooking?*

I set to work. No food had tasted good for months anyway; I'd grown used to chewing and swallowing, chewing and swallowing, like a very morose Pac-man, ignoring my sore throat and total lack of appetite. Doggedly I cut, forked, and chomped. Steadily the meat, carrots, potatoes, and salad disappeared. I left the cookie. Matt didn't eat anything; he'd have something when he got home, he said. He stayed standing, leaning against the wall.

Upon delivering us to this area an hour ago, Nurse No-name had asked me if I wanted some hydroxyzine. Hydroxyzine is a sedative but not a controlled substance, with effects similar to an over-the-counter sleep aid; as such, doctors hand it out freely. Dr. Ortega had prescribed it for me a couple weeks ago when I'd left the rehab center: 20 milligrams, up to three times a day "as needed." Like all the sedatives I'd tried, it had done nothing to help me sleep and rubbed only the slightest edge off the anxiety for a brief spell. Nevertheless, I had been taking it. It was, so Doctor Internet informed me, an anticholinergic, which is a class of drugs that among other effects dampen the signals from inner ear to brain, thereby reducing the discomfort of certain types of vertigo: kind of like a souped-up Dramamine. I'd had hopes it might help *my* type of vertigo, and when it hadn't, another shaky pillar of hope had collapsed. Still, when Nurse No-name asked me if I wanted some hydroxyzine before going down to the ward, I figured I might as well, and when at 6:45 she appeared in the doorway, I thought she was there to dose me.

But no: it turned out she had forgotten about the hydroxyzine and was there to say it was nearly time to go. "They'll take you down in a wheelchair. That's the protocol, sorry." (She didn't look sorry.) "And there'll be a security guard. Protocol. Have you given all your valuables to your husband?" I pulled wallet from purse and handed it to Matt. He already had my rings.

The adrenaline really started to surge when the two men arrived with the wheelchair. Probably one was a nurse and the other the aforementioned security guard, but all I saw were a couple of burly blokes, neither of whom acknowledged me as Nurse No-name pointed to the seat. I sat, and they loaded backpack, purse, and Elephant onto my lap. They swung me around toward the door through which we had come, one of them pushing, the other walking alongside; the side guy swiped his card through the chrome lockbox. They rolled me through, and turned left to face me down a long, bright, empty corridor. I twisted back and saw Matt standing next to No-name. He smiled and called out, "Bye, Bear! See you soon!"

Seized again with anxiety about my stuff, I yelled: "Do you have my wallet?"

"Yes, I have it!"

"Bye!"

"Bye!"

The chair rolled forward, accelerating along the corridor (no no no), making a right turn, a left turn, blank doors sliding by on either side (no no no), ceiling lights fluorescing, the two burly blokes silent, everything silent, warm air smelling of antiseptic, bags a clumsy weight on my lap, turning again, stopping at an elevator (no no no), doors rumbling open, rolling inside, doors rumbling shut (no no no NO), dropping down, down, down the rabbit hole ...

In my life I've known three types of fear: 1) fear of *something*, like the trepidation you feel when you need to give a speech, or your child falls out of a tree and busts her lip, or your plane hits violent turbulence; 2) purely *physical* fear, the electric tide that surges into your gut from nowhere making you think it must be about something until you come to understand it's not about anything, it's just your amygdala's reaction to low blood sugar or hormone shifts or who knows what; 3) fear of *fear itself*, when you dread your own fear so much it becomes a vicious circle, a self-referential loop of panic that worsens the more you try to stop it. Three types of fear, and I'd learned to cope with each by using a mindfulness method: I would, first, notice the feelings— the pounding heart, the dizziness, the tingling skin, the shortness of breath, the intense urge to get up and run. Then I'd acknowledge the feelings, consciously accept them, and carry on doing whatever the occasion demanded, whether that was delivering the speech, driving the child to urgent care, or sitting still in the airplane seat. So far, the method had worked pretty well.

But never, until I was in that wheelchair being taken away to the St. Giles psych ward, had I experienced all three types of fear at once, piling on like football players on a fumble. First, I was quite reasonably afraid of being imprisoned in a cuckoo's nest. Second, my vertigo disorder had months ago flipped a physical switch in my brain to red alert, causing my body to flood day and night with adrenaline. Third and worst of all, my notice-acknowledge-accept strategy had turned into mindfulness run amok: I'd become unable to direct attention away from my own anxiety without that anxiety escalating to an unbearable pitch.

As the elevator doors reopened and the burly blokes rolled me out into another empty corridor, those three fears were feeding on each other, intensifying, spiraling out of control. So, although I remember being pushed down the passage to a dead end with a big white door, I cannot remember let alone describe my mental state. Sane Me had left the building. Mad Me was a speechless, spineless, quivering blob. *"O Oysters," said the Carpenter, "you've had a pleasant run! Shall we be trotting home again?" But answer came there none.*

(Came there none. Came there none. Home again? Home again? Came there none)

I do recall that as the big white door swung open to reveal a small dim room containing a round wooden table and two women in blue scrubs, and I was pushed inside and heard the latch click shut behind me, a voice neither mad nor sane remarked, almost idly:

WHERE IS THE WINDOW, WHERE IS THE VIEW? THIS IS A HOLE, THEY'RE PUTTING US IN A HOLE AND WE'RE NEVER GETTING OUT.

CHAPTER 2

WOOL AND WATER

~~~~~~~~~~~~~~~~~~~~~~~~~

Long ago: a spring morning in 2009, or maybe it was 2010.
The alarm clock *beep-beep-beeps* and I hit Snooze; five minutes later, *beep-beep-beeep*, hit Off, open my eyes, roll onto my back, and stretch. I'm alone in the house. Matt is driving Emily to school; she likes to arrive very early in order to hang out and chat with her middle-school friends. I lounge for a minute, looking at the multicolored book spines in the bookcase, at the Santa Fe sunshine slanting through the blinds, listening to the birds in the lilac bush, thinking about things. What have I got today? No work calls until eight-thirty, so I don't need to rush downstairs to my office juggling tea, toast, and executive presence. Still there is stuff to do, always stuff to do. I press my elbows to the mattress and sit up, yawning, SPINNING *holy shit the room is spinning like a Disneyland teacup* SPIN SPIN SPIN HOLY SHIT!

I throw myself backward, flat to the bed, and lie rigid, staring aghast at the ceiling. Almost immediately the spinning stops. *Don't panic, don't panic, maybe you just sat up too fast. Yeah, that's it, you sat up too fast.* I wait. And wait. Like a toppled statue, for five, six minutes. Then, very slowly, I lever myself up again and …

Everything is normal.

Phew! Well that was weird.

I sit for a while, telling myself I am probably not dying. I've read about vertigo attacks; they're mostly harmless, I've read,

27

but sometimes they can be a sign of something bad: stroke, brain tumor, debilitating inner-ear disorders. My sister-in-law had something wrong with her ears and couldn't keep her balance. What did she have? Somebody's Disease. I can't remember. Anyway, I'm pretty sure I don't have that, whatever it is. If I did, wouldn't I have known about it already? I remove the sheet and blanket to one side and slowly swing my legs off the bed … slowly place my feet on the floor … slowly shift my weight to my feet … slowly rise.

Now I'm standing and everything is fine. *Huh, so bizarre! Glad that's over.* I start to walk around the bed, headed for the bathroom …

(Wait what's this)

The floor is undulating. I stop between bookcase and bed-foot, looking down at the rug, a ten-foot runner with a design of blue, black, and yellow x's: large x's down the middle, little x's down the sides, all on a rust-brown background. I don't *see* the x's moving, and I can balance fine—just as if I were standing on a boat in light seas—but the ground *feels* like it's moving: shifting, swaying, bouncing beneath my feet. The earth has become water. Freaky.

On the other hand, the sensation is familiar. I'm a frequent flyer, and often I've gotten off a plane after a long flight and felt as if I were still aboard, the ground still in motion, in the same way sailors may experience "land-sickness" after disembarking from a sea voyage. "It'll stop soon," my mother would say when I was little, and it always did, so right now I'm not unduly disturbed. I don't feel sick to my stomach, and I figure if I ignore the bouncing it'll go away in a bit, just like the post-flight syndrome. I fix and eat breakfast, descend to the basement office, and work through the morning. When I'm seated, the turbulence increases, which is annoying. But after lunch I walk the dog, and by midafternoon the earth is firm again. Rather than mention it to Emily when she gets home from school or Matt from the college, I chalk up the incident to hormones. With me, everything is hormones; I am 47 and well into perimenopause—which, I have discovered, means a hell of lot more than hot flashes and vaginal dryness.

About a year later the same thing happens, minus the spinning: I simply get out of bed one morning and—Boat World! Once again, I ignore the waves; once again, they calm by midafternoon. I shrug and resign myself to having this thing every now and then. I hate boats, but at least this one doesn't make me vomit, I can walk on it no problem, and it shows up rarely and transiently. I don't like it, but I can handle it; oh yes, I can handle it. It's no big deal.

At some point I come across an article about "benign paroxysmal positional vertigo," or BPPV, which, the article explains, is when tiny calcium crystals (*otochonia*) in one of your inner ear canals dislodge and float around, causing spinning sensations whenever you turn or tilt your head. BPPV is common: 10 to 15 percent of us will have it at some point in our life. The treatment is something called an Epley maneuver, whereby a physical therapist manipulates your body and head in order to tip the ear crystals back into place. Who knew? I decide BPPV must be what I have. Then again, it doesn't exactly sound like me: BPPV makes you dizzy-spinny, not bouncy-rocky, and my thing is definitely bouncy-rocky. Also, BPPV happens only when you move your head, and my thing, when I get it, persists whether I'm in motion or not. In fact, it's at its worst when I'm sitting perfectly still.

In February 2013, a new and equally strange thing happens: a band of pain blooms on the left side of my face, about three inches wide, running from my hairline past my eye down my cheek to my jaw. It's on the surface of the skin, like sunburn, not down in the muscles. Sometimes it tingles or itches. In the mornings I sit at the breakfast table eating shredded wheat and muesli, patting my cheek, wondering what it is, thinking shingles maybe? But there's no rash, no blisters, nothing visible. And isn't shingles supposed to be agonizing? This phenomenon is merely irritating, as if someone had rubbed my cheek with a woolen cloth then kept pressing the cloth to the rubbed patch. My British grandmother insisted "wool next to the skin" was the key to winter warmth. Ugh, itchy! The rubbed-raw feeling hangs around for two or three weeks then goes away.

At my annual physical, I tell Dr. Ortega about the face pain. (I don't mention the bouncy-trouncy vertigo, which hasn't reappeared in a while.) "It does sound like shingles," she says. "Sometimes there aren't any blisters. I'll give you a prescription for the shingles vaccine."

In February 2014, I go to get vaccinated by Oscar, the pharmacist in chief at Del Norte Pharmacy and Medical Supply. The shingles vaccine, he tells me, is a live vaccine, with alive but weakened herpes zoster virus in it (a year later they developed a killed-virus version), so he needs to make sure I'm not having symptoms now. "No, no, I had it last year," I say, rolling up my sleeve while appreciating Oscar's kind eyes and mellow voice. I'm glad I switched from CVS to Del Norte, even though you can't buy moisturizer and shampoo at Del Norte, not unless you want to pay a fortune; they're a *compounding* pharmacy, which as far as I can tell just means *very expensive*. But, they have Oscar. I barely feel the needle.

Sometime in 2015 I get another itchy pain patch, this time on my lower back. Same feeling, like a bad sunburn on top of a moderate bruise. Again, it's invisible; no rash. Again, it lasts a few weeks then dissipates. Maybe, I muse, it came from my pants waistband chafing my skin. Or an allergic reaction to laundry detergent. How could it be shingles, given that I got the vaccine? But Dr. Ortega said it was shingles, so it must be. Vaccines aren't perfect, after all.

I grow used to the rubbed-raw patches and bouncy-ground sensations returning sporadically, never simultaneously, often barely noticeable, seemingly unrelated. They remind me of Alice and the old sheep with the knitting needles in the rowboat: Wool and Water, that chapter is called, Wool and Water. I dislike both wool and water, but I can handle them. Oh yes, I can handle them; they're no big deal.

Several more years go by.

CHAPTER 3

QUEEN OF HEARTS, KNAVE OF HEARTS

~~~~~~~~~~~~~~~~~~~~~~~~~~~~~~~~

D r. Valentine, otolaryngologist, drew a penlight from her pocket. "I'll look in your ears," she said, "but just so you know, with vertigo, 95 percent of the time we can't see anything wrong."

"I understand," I said, not understanding.

The vertigo had returned full force on the night of January 7, 2018. Half-awake at two a.m., in agony from a pulled lower back, I'd rolled onto my left side and, *holy shit wrong wrong WRONG!* screamed my brain, reeling with the worst dizziness I'd ever felt. It stopped when I unrolled, but next morning, hello, there was the ground turbulence: much bouncier than before and, more worrisome, still churning a month later. I made an appointment with PCP Dr. Ortega. She prescribed meclizine (for the seasickness I wasn't having), ordered an antibiotic (for the pain I was, this time down my right cheek radiating deep into my right ear), and referred me to Southwest Ear-Nose-Throat. "I can't see anything in there," she said, "but the ENTs have fancy cameras to look inside your head and see what's going on." Good, I thought, that's what I need, and when the clinic scheduler gave me an appointment with a Dr. Valentine, I was faintly amused: a Queen of Hearts! Who better to chop off my head and poke around inside?

I arrived early for my appointment and asked the tech if it would be all right to remain standing in the exam room while I waited for the doctor. Sitting made the turbulence worse; I felt better upright, swaying side to side or pacing to and fro. But when Dr. Valentine marched in—white-coated, black-pencil-skirted, hair in a bun, sensible heels clicking on the Saltillo tiles—I took a seat, eager for assessment. After all, I thought, I couldn't have expected Dr. Ortega to know about ears. Now, I was with the specialist. Now, I'd get some answers. ENTs encountered vertigo and ear pain all the time, surely, and they had fancy cameras to look inside your head.

As I explained the situation, though, my optimism waned. Dr. Valentine's cold eyes, perfunctory questions, and rapid stomps on the exam chair's foot pedal were a little *too* Queen of Hearts-ish; she seemed totally unimpressed by the oddity of my symptoms and totally unsympathetic to my distress. Having inspected each ear for a few seconds with the penlight, she stepped back. "Yeah, like I said, I can't see anything wrong." She seated herself on the swivel stool and flipped open her laptop.

I didn't expect you to see it with your bare eyes, I thought. Can we move on to the part where you use the fancy cameras and find the cyst, tumor, infection, whatever? A CT scan, I think it's called. I stared at the wall poster displaying the structures of the human ear (anything might go awry in that labyrinth of tiny tubes and coils) and waited for her to continue.

"We just don't know," she said, tap-tapping on her laptop keyboard, "what we're dealing with. We need to do some tests." Good, I thought, now we're getting somewhere. "You'll need a hearing test and a VNG test. The hearing test we can do today. The VNG test, that's when we test the function of your inner ears, that takes a few weeks to schedule."

I knew about VNG tests. A friend of mine had had terrible vertigo and was sent for one. She said it was bad: they put goggles on her and flashed lights in her eyes, she said, and squirted hot and cold water in her ears, and she got crazy dizzy. Maybe, I consoled myself, they'd do the CT scan first and find the problem, and then I wouldn't have to undergo the scary VNG.

"… so let's get these tests done and we can go from there. Any questions?"

(Wait, did she mention a CT? I didn't hear her say CT) "Um, OK, but don't you want to do some kind of, I don't know—imaging?"

"We can refer you for a CT at the hospital later, if it's necessary. We don't have the equipment to do them here. First we should do these tests. Go from there."

"I see." (So you *don't* actually have fancy cameras. Lies, all lies)

"Also, I can refer you to physical therapy. They're right downstairs. Would you like physical therapy?"

"Um … I guess so. Sure."

I must have looked upset, because she swiveled on her stool to face me and said in a poor-baby tone, "I know it's miserable, feeling dizzy and sick all the time."

"Well, yes. It's pretty bad."

"You know what? Lemme get some of that wax out of your ears."

"Oh, OK. That'd be nice."

She rustled up a water syringe, pink plastic catch bowl and stainless-steel picks, yanked on a pair of pink latex gloves, and dug in. *Eek … ack … oog … ew … aaahhh.*

Smiling in mutually repulsed satisfaction, we gazed at the sticky brown goo on the tissue. Then, with an air of that's-enough-fun-for-today, the Queen disposed of the tissue, peeled off the gloves, picked up her laptop while snapping the lid shut, and turned to face me: "Great, so we'll get you those tests, go from there. Hearing test and VNG—you can schedule them both at the reception desk. I'll see you again once we have the results. PT is downstairs."

"OK, thank you."

"Have a good week." Out she marched, heels clicking.

I gathered my purse and my already-fat medical file folder and made the short walk to the schedulers' desk. Boing, boing, boing went the floor. There was a line. As I waited my turn, swaying gently side to side—*get the tests, go from there, get the tests, go from there*—I thought about the Queen of Hearts' attempt at empathy: "I know it's miserable, feeling dizzy and sick all the time." The attempt had failed. Why?

Before becoming a writer, I'd spent 25 years with a company that offered corporate training in leadership, sales, and customer service skills. Among many other lessons, I'd learned that when you work with agitated customers there is a paramount rule: *Attend to feelings first, facts second.* Confronted with a scared, angry, or upset person, you should address the emotions of the situation *before* you address the practicalities. Start by explaining the plan, and the upset person won't hear you; start by acknowledging their upset, however briefly, and they may relax enough to discuss the plan. Like many doctors I was to encounter on my journey through Madland, Dr. Valentine had ignored (or more likely, had never been taught) the feelings-before-facts rule. She left the feelings too late; moreover, she got the feelings wrong, for I'd told her explicitly that I did *not* feel dizzy or sick, just that I was constantly on a boat. In jumping to the facts, she overlooked my feelings. As a result, I did not trust her.

I did, however, sympathize. Her flat voice when she'd said, "With vertigo, 95 percent of the time we can't see anything wrong" spoke of a specialty steeped in futility, rife with complaints physicians could do little about. The blank looks of Dr. Ortega, and now Dr. Valentine, told me that vertigo was largely a medical mystery: mechanisms ill-understood, drugs ineffective, cures nonexistent. Treatments? There was, I would come to find, meclizine for queasiness, diuretics to dry up eustachian tubes, physical maneuvers to coax wayward ear crystals back into place, and, if your inner-ear nerves were damaged to the point where you couldn't balance, exercises to encourage your brain to adapt. That was about it. With such a limited set of options (not even the ability to order people's heads removed!) no wonder the Queen of Hearts was grumpy. Must be a drag, I thought as I took a bouncy step closer to the schedulers' desk, to be a doctor and the most helpful thing you do in a morning is to scoop out somebody's earwax.

A week later I returned for my PT appointment with Dr. Cook. The room had a polished cement floor dotted with exercise mats, nerf balls, and small orange traffic cones. A high, cushioned table stood against one wall; some clear plastic hula-hoops leaned against another wall; and in the far corner, a metal desk bore stacks of journals, a computer, and decks of playing cards. The place seemed to me a mashup of medical office, yoga studio, and doggy daycare.

Dr. Cook looked to be in his early 40s, with a slim build, balding pate, and black-rimmed Harry Potter glasses. He wore a bright red shirt. Maybe it was the shirt and the hula hoops and the playing cards, or maybe it was the memory of Dr. Valentine; in any case, the Knave of Hearts came to mind. Standing by his desk, he glanced through the questionnaire I'd filled out in the waiting area, then looked up with friendly energy: "So, tell me about your vertigo!"

I had been seized, I said, with extreme dizziness upon rolling over in the middle of the night of January seventh, and since then I'd felt I was on a boat: no nausea, no problems balancing, worse when I'm sitting still, not so bad when I walk, goes away when I'm driving or riding in a car. I described the attacks of maybe-shingles on both sides of my head and speculated that those attacks had caused inner-ear damage, which in turn was causing the vertigo. I told him I had tried doing Epley maneuvers at home, guided by YouTube videos, to no avail. I mentioned the hearing test I'd completed.

"Yes, I have your hearing test results," he said, taking a clipboard from the desk and flipping through the pages. "No problems there. Your hearing is a lot better than mine, ha-ha! Well, let's check out a few things. Have a seat"—he pulled out a light chair, placing it in the middle of the room—"sorry, I know you said sitting was the most uncomfortable!"

"No, no, that's OK," I said, encouraged by his forthright manner and by the sense that he, unlike Dr. Valentine, had been listening. *Feelings first, facts second. Good job, Knave.*

He seated himself before me and proceeded to lead me through a battery of exercises: Move head side to side, up and down. Close eyes and touch my nose with a finger, open them and touch his finger with my finger, follow his moving finger with my eyes. Tilt, look, turn, close, open, touch. "Any dizziness?" he kept asking. "No," I kept saying, "but I still feel like I'm on a boat." Next, he said he was going to hold my head and snap it fast from side to side. *Eek!* But again: no dizziness. He had me stand up and balance on one foot, balance on both feet with eyes closed, balance while standing on a foam mat with eyes closed (that was hard), walk to and fro on a diagonal—*ok girls, line up let's do piqué turns across the floor*—walk and turn quickly, walk and stop suddenly. He had me sit down again, brought over an orange traffic cone, placed it on the floor before me, and asked me to lean forward and pick it up.

"Any dizziness?"

"Nope."

I felt proud as I passed each test, but I could also see that passing the tests was giving a possibly undesirable impression: I could balance fine, and I was neither stumbling nor pausing, so what was my problem? The Knave of Hearts' eyes held a scintilla of frost as he pushed back his chair and said, "Tell me how it *feels.*"

"Like I'm on a boat."

"You mean, like the ground is moving? Like water?"

"Yes. Just like on a boat." *Christ, how many times must I say it?* I tried another metaphor: "It's like the floor is sort of elastic. Bouncing up and down."

"When do you feel it?"

"All the time. Bouncing and rocking. Sometimes it's like I'm tipping back and forth or sliding down a wave. It never stops, well, it stops when I'm driving a car, but that's the only time. Oh, and it's better when I'm sitting in a rocking chair."

"Because you can rock to the same rhythm?"

"I guess … there isn't really a rhythm, though. It's like being on a b-… on the ocean."

"Hmm. Have you noticed when it's worse or better?"

"Yes. Basically it's bad in the mornings and improves as the day goes on. It's best at about five p.m. Gets worse after dinner and before bed." (Storm demons attack at night)

"I see," said the Knave. "In the past month, have you bumped your head at all?"

I thought back. "No."

"Are you sure? Maybe you stepped off a curb and jarred your spine?"

I thought some more. "No. Really, I haven't. Oh, I did throw my back out. It's fine now."

"Hmm. Have you been on a cruise ship recently?"

"Ha-ha, no. I'd never go on a cruise. I hate boats."

"Any changes to medications?"

"Yes." I launched into tales of hormones. Once it had become clear that the turbulence wasn't going away this time, I'd raced to Dr. Ortega's nurse practitioner and had her switch me from estrogen pills to an estrogen skin patch plus oral progesterone. The patch, which provides a steadier infusion than oral estrogen, helped my mood but did nothing for the vertigo. The oral progesterone, however, definitely *did* help the vertigo, which was lucky, because I took it before bed. One time I forgot, and the mattress rocked and rolled until I remembered, got up, and took the little round shiny orange pill.

"… Anyway," I said, "I don't know why the oral progesterone helps, but it does. Why do you suppose it helps?"

Dr. Cook was flipping through my chart again. "Interesting! I don't know!" he said, putting the clipboard aside. "So, here's what I think is going on. You've got something called benign paroxysmal positional vertigo, or BPPV." He picked up two of the clear plastic hula-hoops and hoisted them at perpendicular angles, saying, "These are two of your three inner ear canals. The little balls"—inside each hoop was a clump of colored pellets—"are calcium crystals, also known as otochonia, which are supposed to stay lodged in a pocket, but sometimes, like for instance if you bump your head, the crystals can get dislodged into the canals"—he tipped the hoops, causing the pellets to swirl around—"like this, which creates a spinning sensation."

"Yes, I know about BPPV, but I don't …"

"Right, you don't feel any spinning. But"—he raised an index finger, like Poirot revealing the solution to a murder mystery, and his voice grew hushed with triumph—"I have seen a *few* patients with BPPV who feel as if they are *rocking*, not spinning!"

Amazed relief was clearly the reaction expected, so I obliged him: "Really? Wow!"

"It's true! So let's go in the other room, and we'll do some Epley maneuvers."

"Oh, OK. I did try to do those at home, but I probably didn't do them right."

"Yes, well, don't feel bad. They're hard to do on your own."

I stood up to follow him, then hesitated. "Um, I'm just wondering, what about nerve damage? I've read that the shingles virus, if it's on your head, can damage your ear nerves."

"No." As definite as a mallet striking a croquet ball. "If you had vestibular neuritis, you'd be falling all over the place. You couldn't even walk."

"I see, but if it was just minor damage, wouldn't—"

"Come on back this way."

The collar of his red shirt preceded me into a smaller room with an examining table, on which he instructed me to sit. I was feeling a touch scared; all the YouTube videos of PTs performing Epley maneuvers showed the patient getting intensely dizzy, if only for a minute or two. I was game, though. Anything to get this fixed.

Here's how an Epley maneuver works: You sit on a surface with your legs stretched out. Behind you is a pillow placed so that when you lie back it's beneath your shoulders, not your head. While you're sitting up, the PT has you turn your head 45 degrees to left or right (depending on which ear he thinks is affected), supports your head with his hand, then lowers you back *fast*—almost like doing a backward dive—so that your neck is craned down and to the side, head dropped lower than your shoulders. If anyone wanted to slit your throat, you'd be in the ideal position for it; they'd have ample opportunity, too, because you stay that way for about a minute. Then, without lifting your head, you rotate your head to the right, again to a 45-degree angle, and hold that pose. Next you roll onto your side and assume a fetal position: knees curled, chin tucked. You stay there for one more minute and finally sit up, your legs hanging off the side of the table. The purpose of these moves is to coax the ear crystals back into the pocket, like in one of those maddening tip-the-teensy-marbles-into-the-holes games.

Throughout the procedure you must keep your eyes open, because the PT is watching your eyeballs. Somebody watching your eyeballs is very different from somebody gazing into your eyes; the latter can feel romantic, while the former feels disconcertingly lab-rattish. As Dr. Cook took me through the

Epleys—first on the left side, then on the right, then left again, then right again—he was watching my eyes for something called *nystagmus*: quick jerking motions that happen when your vision system is trying desperately to match the sensations of movement being conveyed by your inner ear. Imagine holding your head still while counting the horses on an exceptionally fast merry-go-round: *Horse, horse, horse* and *jerk, jerk, jerk* go your eyeballs.

As Dr. Cook stared at (not into) my eyes, he was also asking me what I was feeling. I'd been nervous at the prospect of wild dizziness, but it turned out my fears were needless. After he flipped me back the first time, I felt nothing unusual for maybe ten seconds; then a wave hit me, which I reported: "Oof, there's a big dip!" Then nothing again, except the same old continuous, mild turbulence, punctuated occasionally by a more dramatic whoosh. Dr. Cook kept on staring at my eyeballs as I went through the paces: flip back, hold the pose, turn head, hold the pose, fetal position, hold the pose, sit up. Repeat. Repeat. Repeat.

Finally, after the fourth maneuver, he said we were done. "Interesting!" he said. "You've got nystagmus on *both* sides! Very slight eye jerks, barely noticeable, but definitely there."

"Both sides? Really?"

"Yes, both sides, although it's a little more pronounced on the right."

I was gratified to know that someone had been able to detect an outward physical marker, however minor, of my hitherto invisible ailment, and pleased to think I had learned a technique that might help.

"So, how often should I do these Epley maneuvers?" I asked. "Twice a day? Three times a day?"

The Knave of Hearts smirked like a magician bringing an elaborate card trick to a satisfying finish. "Nope, that's it! You're all set!"

"I am?"

"Yup! You're done!"

"Oh … OK, great!"

Then why are we still on the boat?

————

Maybe it takes a day or two for the Epleys to kick in, I mused as I walked the aisles of Office Depot half an hour later looking for poster board for a work project. Maybe the ear crystals are back in the pocket, but the effects linger. Yeah, that's it … the effects linger.

The effects were doing more than lingering, though; they had gotten worse. The floor of Office Depot was undulating vigorously, the shelves of pens, tape, and notebooks wobbling on either side of me. It was like being in an extremely unfun version of an inflatable bouncy castle.

Yet I still had no difficulty balancing. If you ask me why, all I can say is, one, most people can balance on a boat once they get their sea legs, and two, I have better balance than most people. In my dancing days, double pirouettes on a raked stage were a basic expectation, and I'd held onto that fine equilibrium into middle age. Today, when I tell a doctor I have chronic vertigo, he invariably asks me, "Any falls?" and appears mildly surprised when I say No, no falls, not even a half-fall, not even the threat of a fall. I can almost see the cursor clicking *close* on the Serious Condition file in his mind. After all, if the patient isn't throwing up or falling down, why worry? No loss of function, no problem, right?

Wrong. Here's the problem: Being on a boat, when you're *not* on a boat, is terrifying.

I found the poster board, traversed the heaving floor to the checkout counter, and paid, hoping the clerk couldn't perceive my discombobulation. Driving home, I noted again how the waves went away entirely while the car was in motion but resurged whenever I stopped at a red light: Stop. Wait. Boing, boing, boing. Green light, drive on, no more boings. When I had to check my blind spot, I did it gingerly, afraid that twists and turns of the head might disorient me, but they didn't seem to make any difference. My dizziness was neither paroxysmal nor positional. Yet the Knave of Hearts had seemed very sure it was BPPV, and that he had fixed it.

That evening after dinner I went to the basement office, curled up on the couch with the nubbly beige slipcover (the Magicouch, I called it, because I'd found it offered a near-magical cure for occasional insomnia, something about having my back pressed against the cushions) and googled "dizziness persisting after Epley maneuver." Up popped a discussion forum with dozens of posts, mostly from women, some talking about BPPV but others talking about this weird up-and-down sensation that Epleys did not mitigate. I scrolled along until one thread caught my eye: "It's like walking on a trampoline," someone commented. "Omg it's the worst," replied someone else, "yesterday I took a step, and the floor went up to my neck."

Walking on a trampoline? Floor up to the neck? They were describing my thing precisely! I read further and saw that many commenters were using the same name for it: *vestibular migraine.* I'd never had a migraine headache in my life; nevertheless, I clutched at the term like a hot cup of tea on a cold morning. Even if vestibular migraine wasn't what I had, clearly there existed more types of vertigo than I'd been told of. There was information to hunt down.

————

Over the next two weeks I read up on dizziness-and-balance disorders, mostly on internet sites but also in a few scientific journals. Balance, I learned, is a matter of inputs from three sources: your eyes, your inner ears, and something called *proprioception,* also known as self-sensing—the information the muscles and bones of the body convey to the brain about their position in space. When signals from eyes, ears, and muscles are in sync and functioning properly, your cerebellum, the part of the brain responsible for balance, interprets the world as normal and steady. When the signals are out of whack—say, because of nerve damage or too much pressure in an ear canal—you may feel dizzy.

Dizziness is a general term that encompasses light-headedness, vertigo, and loss of balance. *Vertigo* is a false sense of motion (usually spinning, but sometimes rocking, bouncing, or falling) that may be caused by vestibular problems. *Vestibular* refers to the vestibules, or tubes, of the inner ear. The *vestibular nerve* is the pair of big cranial nerves that carry sensory impulses from inner ears to brain. *Vestibular migraine* is a dysfunction of the vestibular nerve; it often causes vertigo rather than a headache. *Vestibular neuritis* or *labyrinthitis* is an inflammation of the tiny nerves or tissues of the inner ear.

By the time I went for physical therapy round two with the Knave of Hearts, my skin pain and earache had gone away; the bouncy vertigo remained, however, and because I was even more certain it was all down to the shingles virus, I was determined to be treated for vestibular neuritis. A physician friend had told me that shingles on the head can cause damage to the facial nerve, which in turn may cause any number of awful symptoms: facial paralysis, hearing loss, tinnitus, and/or vertigo. Whether the damage was on my left or right side, or both, and whether the vestibular nerve was also somehow involved, I did not know. All I knew (or *thought* I knew) was that I'd had several shingles attacks, two of them on my head, which had affected the nerves of one or both ears, which were now sending messed-up signals to my brain. I also knew that although damaged nerves can't be repaired, the brain is good at adapting to messed-up signals, and special exercises can encourage it to adapt. I wanted to learn those exercises.

The Knave was happy to oblige. On my second visit to his yoga doggy daycare studio, after I told him the Epleys hadn't worked and that even though I could walk I thought the problem really might be vestibular neuritis, he took an ace of diamonds from a card pack on his desk, sat me down, and showed me how to hold the card out and move it left and right, over and over, while simultaneously shaking my head "no" in the opposite direction with eyes glued to the ace. Next I had to move the card up and down while nodding "yes" and keeping eyes glued. I was to do these exercises five times a day, first sitting then standing, for about five minutes each time. Ideally, he said, I'd make myself a little dizzy but not a lot dizzy: "maybe a three out of ten," he said, "and remember, it's how often you do it, not how long you do it."

Then he demonstrated how to perform Epley maneuvers on my own. I could tell his money was still on the roving ear crystals, where my money was not, but I figured it couldn't hurt to learn. He stretched himself out on the platform table and showed me how I should use a pillow thick enough only to crane my head back slightly. "You don't need to strain," he said. "The most important thing is to hold each position for at least a minute and *don't lift your head* when you turn it from one side to the other." He was a good demonstrator, and when I left I felt confident I could replicate the moves. He also let me keep the ace of diamonds.

For the next two weeks I did the eye exercises faithfully, five times (OK, sometimes four times) a day, working up to where I could do them while raised on the balls of my feet and with my thumb instead of the card as a focal point. Tedious, but not difficult. For good measure I also did Epleys several times a week, both sides, following the Knave's directions with care.

It was now late March, spring break was over, and Emily had returned to college in Ohio. Matt was around as usual, trundling back and forth to campus, looking forward to the end of his run as dean. I made us dinner most nights. During the day I worked on my third leadership book, sometimes downstairs at my desk but mostly sitting in the rocking chair at the dining room table. I walked the dog and did the occasional ballet barre. The vertigo stayed about the same.

But not exactly the same. Ever since I'd rolled over in the wee hours of January seventh, triggering this whole episode, I'd been unable to lie on my left side without feeling horribly dizzy. The good news was that now, with April approaching, I'd become capable of doing it—lying on my left side, that is—as long as I kept my head propped high on two pillows. Moreover, although the ground was still very bouncy in the morning and evening, it was definitely less bouncy in the late afternoon. I noticed that cutting back on sugar helped. And the bedtime pro-gesterone still worked to placate the storm demons so I could go to sleep. Baby steps, I thought, baby steps. The eye exercises must be doing something.

I still hunted for clues on the internet. One evening while reclining on the Magicouch, laptop on lap, I came across an arti-cle on the website of a Dr. Legg, a dizziness-and-balance special-ist based in Chicago. The topic was a rare disorder called Mal de Débarquement Syndrome. *Mal de débarquement* is French for land-sickness, which, you may recall, is when you get off a boat and feel as if you're still aboard with the deck moving beneath your feet: in English, "sickness of disembarking." When such sickness lingers beyond a few hours or days, in some cases con-tinuing for months, that is Mal de Débarquement Syndrome—MdDS or "mal debarquement" for short. In most cases it occurs after a stint of travel and is thought to arise from the brain get-ting "stuck" in an adaptive pattern. The hallmark of MdDS, Dr. Legg wrote, is a bouncing or rocking sensation that does *not* cause nausea and that goes *away* when the patient is in a state of passive motion; for example, riding in a car. The typical sufferer is a 40- to 60-year-old woman who has been on an ocean cruise.

By now I was sitting upright, transfixed. This was me! Well, except for the ocean cruise part. But otherwise, me! I raced onward, hoping to read of treatments ...

"There are no established treatments for MdDS."

Damn.

"Typically, symptoms gradually subside over months or, in some cases, years."

Years? Are you kidding me?

"Benzodiazepines, such as Valium, are the only medication proven to reduce symptoms."

No thank you. Not taking addictive drugs.

"One experimental treatment has shown limited promise. Developed by Drs. Cranker and Wanker of Tallahassee, Florida, it involves strapping the patient to a chair in a small circular windowless room and spinning them around while they stare at black-and-white stripes projected on the wall rotating the opposite way, and then …"

Ha-ha-ha oh my god stop it!

"It is interesting to note that MdDS patients are often post-menopausal women on hormone replacement therapy (HRT). There may be a link to fluctuating hormone levels …"

Hmm. That is indeed interesting.

"… so, these patients may want to go off their HRT."

Wait, what? Go OFF it? That doesn't follow at all!

"Although function typically remains high, MdDS can negatively affect quality of life."

No shit, my dude.

"In general, the best prescription is 'tincture of time' combined with methods that help the patient reduce vigilance."

Tincture of time and reduced vigilance, eh? In other words, tell the silly old hags to go home and relax. Great, that's just great.

To be fair, Dr. Legg put it all much more professionally. And, albeit disheartening, his article had supplied my first real sense that somebody, somewhere, knew what I was coping with. My follow-up appointment with Dr. Valentine was in a few days. I was armed with a name.

"Oh, sure, I know about mal debarquement, but I've never heard of it happening without travel." The Queen of Hearts was ensconced once again on her swivel stool, black pencil skirt stretched over her crossed legs, white coat crisp. She was giving me some impressive side-eye.

"Um, yeah …" I was on my feet, swaying to and fro as usual, riding the boat deck. "… from what I've read, I guess 20 percent of cases are non-travel-related."

"Huh. Have you had the VNG test yet?"

"No, I rescheduled it for next week."

"Fine. Once we get the results of the VNG, we can go from there. Any falls?"

"No."

"How's the ear pain?"

"Gone."

"Good. You've been seeing Dr. Cook for PT?"

"Yes, I'm seeing him again tomorrow. Are there any treatments for this thing?"

"Just PT." She typed furiously. "Well, at least now we have a name for it. I'm sure the PT will help." She snapped her laptop shut, made to exit, turned back with a frown. "Have a good week."

————

The Knave of Hearts was leaning over his desk, peering at my chart on his computer monitor.

"Does it say, 'Crazy lady thinks this is mal debarquement'?" I asked. "Ha-ha."

He chuckled. "No, it doesn't say that." Then, straightening up to face me: "To be honest, mal debarquement did occur to me when I first saw you, only there hadn't been any travel!"

"Right, I guess in 20 percent of cases, it's non-travel-related."

"Huh. Are the eye exercises doing anything?"

"I can't tell. They don't make me dizzy at all. And the vertigo seems a bit better, but it's still there. Like, all the time."

"Ah. Yeah, they're not doing anything, then. Unfortunately, there's hardly any research on mal debarquement, because it's so rare. I don't know much about it, honestly. You'd need to see an expert. Like that guy in Chicago you mentioned, Dr. Legg, he's the main guy—hey, I'm actually going to a conference next week in Chicago where he'll be speaking!"

"Oh, cool!" I did think it was kind of cool. But not all that cool.

"Anyway, here's what I think happened: You had BPPV"—his eyes widened behind his Harry Potter glasses—"and the BPPV *triggered* the mal debarquement!"

His dedication to the BPPV theory was becoming annoying. Most doctors, I was starting to see, are hedgehogs, not foxes: they know one big thing, the thing they can fix, and they'll stick to that one big thing come what may. Few are the intrepid diagnosticians who maintain fox mind, digging, digging through the evidence until they've solved the case. Few doctors have the time for fox mind. Still, I had by now developed my own theory of how mal debarquement works, and I shared it, tentatively:

"I think the reason mal debarquement is so hard to adapt to," I said, "is that it *is* the adaptation. It's the brain's way of interpreting bizarre ear signals in a way that keeps you from feeling sick or losing your balance. It interprets them as something normal, something it knows, like being on a boat or car or plane. That's why those eye exercises to help my brain adapt don't do any good. As far as my brain is concerned, it's already adapting."*

The Knave seemed neither convinced nor particularly interested.

He taught me a few new exercises geared to improving proprioception—that is, sensing more accurately where my body was in space—but "they probably won't have much effect," he said. He opined that my symptoms would likely go away "with

---

* This theory, I now believe, is essentially correct. A fuller explanation appears in Chapter 11.

time." He said I did not need to undergo the VNG goggles-lights-water-squirts test (*yay*), because for me, there was no purpose to it. And he reiterated that Valium was the only drug known to help mal debarquement—that and amitriptyline, an old-time antidepressant often used to treat migraines.

"I've taken amitriptyline for my own migraines," he said with a mournful shrug. "Gave me the most awful hallucinations."

Hallucinations?!? Alrighty, then. Tincture of time it is.

———

In the second week of April I flew to Austin, Texas, to visit an old friend for a few days. I had hesitated when buying my plane ticket, worried that my condition would have turned aluminum sky-tubes from merely unpleasant to full-on harrowing, but as I towed my roller bag across the red brick tiled floor of the Albuquerque Sunport, I noticed the vertigo was less bad. Then, when I sat down at the gate to wait for boarding, I noticed the vertigo was … nearly gone! In Austin, the ground held steady, and my friend and I had fun. I wondered if the improvement was a matter of being at a lower altitude; when I returned home to the Santa Fe mountains, however, I was still on terra firma, and there I stayed for more than two years. Oh, the sea came in from time to time, sometimes choppy, sometimes light, rocking me for an hour or a week, but never intolerably so. The nerve pain, too, went dormant. Tincture of time had worked.

For Christmas of 2018, my in-laws came to visit. In May 2019, Emily graduated from college, our dear old dog had to be put to sleep, and my third leadership book came out. In November 2019, I finished the manuscript of my first novel. Toward the end of January 2020, my two brothers and I flew to Philadelphia where we said goodbye to our mother, dying of heart disease, and moved our father into the memory care ward of the assisted living facility.

In April 2020, the Covid pandemic shut down New Mexico.

Through all this I enjoyed calm waters, sanguinely unaware that the storm demons were not defeated but merely fallen back. On the morning of July sixteenth, their strength regathered, they struck again—hard.

CHAPTER 4

ADVICE FROM CATERPILLARS

M y goodness, Jocelyn, your heart is racing a mile a minute!"
I shrugged. "Yeah, my heart rate is always kinda fast.
And like I said, the vertigo is bad."

Dr. Ortega's nurse practitioner (a new one) lowered her
stethoscope, placed a hand on my upper back, and rubbed.
"Gosh, you're just a nervous girl, aren't you?!"

"Ha-ha! I guess I am." *We prefer Nervous Well-known Author,
but sure, whatever.*

"Do you know about deep breathing?"

"Um … yes? I do know about deep breathing."

"Slow, deep breaths: they'll relax you. You definitely haven't
had a stroke. Now, you mentioned hormones. Where do you get
these hormones?" Her brow furrowed with suspicion.

"Uh … from Dr. Ortega." I gestured to the wall: *Your boss,
who sits in that office there.*

"Oh. Well, you can't just chase the hormones, you know.
Because they fluctuate. The levels go up and down."

"I understand." *Yes, we know what fluctuate means.*

"You need to be taking supplements, getting exercise, eating
healthy."

"I understand."

"I actually don't prescribe hormones for my patients."

"Ah." *Then it's a good thing we're not your patient, isn't it?*

We engaged in a brief stare-down. Nurse Just-a-Nervous-Girl flinched first. "OK, well, I'll give you these prescriptions for a month and we can see how it goes. Estradiol patch, 0.1 milligram, and you wanted to switch from the norethindrone back to the progesterone?"

"Yes, please." *Write the scripts! Write them or I'll strangle you with a stethoscope!*

She wrote the scripts while I breathed deeply. I drove to CVS (alas, my insurance had forced me to abandon Del Norte, home of the charming Oscar) and picked up the meds.

The Santa Fe summer of 2020 was chugging along hot, dry, and virus-laden. A few days ago I'd woken up feeling a bit off, sweaty, head a bit swimmy. Thinking nothing of it, I sat up, and, bloody hell, the room SPUN, just as it had on that morning a decade ago, only harder. This time, though, I knew what to do: I tossed off two Epleys, one on each side as taught by the Knave of Hearts, then lay quietly on my back until the spinning ceased. I sat up again. The spinning resumed. I lay down once more, waited a longer time, and sat up to more spinning. I did another Epley, sat up—more spinning. *Goddammit!* I got out of bed, stumbled, grabbed onto the windowsill, and tried desperately not to fall as the world continued to revolve.

In fifteen seconds or so the revolutions stopped, leaving behind my old friend The Boat. *OK, OK, you got this; it's no big deal.* I went to the kitchen where Matt was slicing a banana and gave an incident report; he hugged me and told me to go lie down, he'd bring me some tea.

Reaching for the mug, I realized I couldn't roll onto my side—my right side, this time—without feeling unbearably dizzy. *What an incredible drag. But you got this. Keep moving.*

Matt didn't have any classes to teach that day, so later in the morning we walked downtown to pick up my watch, which had been having its battery replaced at a small shop near the Plaza. Then we went to one of the hotels for lunch on the patio; due to

Covid, all the restaurant seating in town was outdoors. The sun was strong, the tourists few. I had been in fairly good spirits since finding that walking was, as before, bouncy but not difficult; as I ingested my chicken enchiladas, however, I noticed that the boat had added some crazy new tilts to its bounce. I felt as though I were constantly sliding down a wave in one direction or another, and objects kept blurring, mildly but unpleasantly, before my eyes. I said nothing to Matt about these new plot twists. It had happened before, I reminded myself; yes, it did seem worse this time, but it had happened before, had faded away, and no doubt would fade away again. Besides, I was pretty sure I knew the reason for it: I had been cutting back on my HRT. I was down to a very low dose on the estradiol patch and had switched to a different progestin, norethindrone instead of progesterone, all of which, I thought ruefully, had probably been a mistake. I would make an appointment with Dr. Ortega, get the hormones read-justed, and I'd be back in business.

Dr. Ortega's scheduler gave me a choice of nurse practi-tioner tomorrow or Dr. Ortega never. But that was fine, because Nurse Practitioner Just-a-Nervous-Girl coughed up the Rx for the stronger estradiol patch, which I slapped onto my tummy with good hope. Even after a fortnight with no improvement to the vertigo, I wasn't worried; even when I began waking up in a sweat, even when adrenaline started to buzz in my gut at intervals throughout the day, even when the itchy pain returned all over my scalp, even when breathing at night seemed a bit difficult. *Patience, patience above all.* I knew from experience it could take six weeks for the estrogen to take full effect, and that my body needed time to adjust to the different progestin. "So annoying," I said to my friend Susan in Toronto. "I wish the hor-mones worked faster, but there we go. Nothing to do but wait."

"Is there any chance it's Covid?" Susan wondered. "You sound kinda hoarse."

"Oh, no, I don't think so. I don't have *bad* shortness of breath or a sore throat or cough or anything like that. It's just this weird thing of mine. I'll be fine."

I was still sleeping soundly, eight hours a night. I was tired during the day, though—chronic vertigo is exhausting—so I'd usually take a short nap after lunch. I'd always been a champion napper, able to fall asleep on sofas, on planes, in other people's living rooms, sitting up, lying down, wherever. As a small child, I'd never minded having to nap: upstairs I'd go to my bed, read a comic book for a while or listen to a record on the record player, then snuggle down with Old Ticket and New Ticket (my stuffed elephants of yore) and drift off within moments. To me, napping was the ultimate balm for sorrows and fears.

So at 1:30 p.m. on August the first, when I stretched out with head propped on three pillows, book in hand, it was in the untroubled expectation that I would be enjoying another pleasant siesta. No, I couldn't lie on my right side or my stomach, but on my back was fine. Hey, I'm Thomas Jefferson, I thought, recalling the Monticello tour with Matt during which we'd viewed Jefferson's bed and the guide had pointed out the angled headboard, informing us that men of the era considered a raised torso to be the healthiest sleep position. I read for five or ten minutes. Then, feeling drowsy, I laid the book aside, folded my hands across my stomach, closed my eyes, and relaxed into the soporific mist. Floating ... sinking ... dreaming ...

NO SLEEP!!!

Gasp, head jerk, eyes flying open. *What the fuck?! What the ... OK, OK, no worries, it's just that thing that happens when you're falling asleep and your leg spasms. Try again, now. Sleep mode. That's it. Sleep mode.* I recomposed myself with eyes closed.

Half an hour later, I gave up. A switch in my brain had flipped, I'd *felt* it flip, to Red Alert, Brace for Incoming, House on Fire. The nap, once my safe space, was now a danger zone.

But plenty of people can't nap in the day, I thought as I awaited Dr. Greene's call. They do fine. I was fine! After all, I was still sleeping at night—sort of. I'd been trying different regimens with the hormones. The orange Skittles (progesterone) calmed the vertigo better than the white Tic-Tacs (norethindrone) and helped me fall asleep, but the Skittles had the unfortunate effect of wearing off dramatically at three a.m., causing me to wake up in a cold sweat followed by violent shaking. When I switched back to the Tic-Tacs, I found they had weaker effects for worse and for better: I had a harder time falling asleep and still woke up at three a.m., but minus the sweats and shakes. Most nights I'd leave Matt asleep in our room and Emily in hers—she was home from grad school for the first part of August—and tip-toe downstairs to the Magicouch, which at this stage still held some of its soporific power. I'd be awake for an hour or two but eventually would drift off with head propped high, back pressed against the nubbly slipcovered cushions, and snooze till seven or eight a.m. I was keeping a sleep diary: as I calculated it, I was getting maybe six hours a night, which didn't seem too bad. Pretty good, in fact ... if only I could nap.

Thinking it might be wise to get another round of physical therapy, I called Southwest ENT only to be informed that Dr. Cook, a.k.a. the Knave of Hearts, had moved to Albuquerque, and that they weren't taking vertigo patients anyway. Most area doctors in this time of Covid had shifted their practice to telemedicine, making hands-on care inaccessible. Turning to Google, I found a Dr. Greene, who advertised himself as a hearing and balance specialist, and read a few of his reviews: "caring ... responsive ... expert." I called his office and booked a phone visit. At the appointed time I seated myself in the rocking chair, eyes glued to my phone screen, notepad at the ready. After a short wait, the ringtone sounded. *Now remember: alert, cooperative!*

"Hello, Dr. Greene, thank you so much for calling!"

He seemed nice, making sympathetic noises as I explained the situation: bouncy castle, insomnia, etcetera. When I mentioned the beneficial effects of the progesterone, however, he broke in with a tone of surprise: "How did you figure *that* out?"

"How did I—I don't know," I stammered. "By observation? I've just noticed it helps. Also I've read that oral progesterone has a metabolite that acts on the brain like a benzodiazepine, which makes sense since Valium is the one drug that's been shown to—"

"Right, right. OK, so, based on what you've told me, an MRI will be the first step. First we rule out the really bad stuff, then we can look at other things."

Though I'd been bracing for it, the word *MRI* made my innards do a sick flop. Not because I was afraid of finding "the really bad stuff" (translation: brain tumor)—at this point it would have been a relief just to know my symptoms had a concrete cause—but because I was deathly afraid of MRI machines. CT machines, I had convinced myself, were fine because they were big and open, like giant donuts, but MRI machines were definitely not fine because they were narrow, dark tubes into which they slid you and left you sealed up like a vampire in a coffin where no one could hear you scream. Or so I imagined. Still, I had heard about the newer "open" MRIs and "wide bore" MRIs, and I figured there had to be one of those in Santa Fe. I shoved the MRI worries aside and tuned in again to Dr. Greene.

"Now, the other thing I want you to do is look up vestibular dot org. It's a very informative website and it will give you a lot of information about the various types of vertigo."

I had discovered that site myself two years ago, but it had probably been updated since then, so, good suggestion, good suggestion. I thanked him and wrote "vestibular.org" on my notepad. "Can I ask," I continued, "do *you* think what I have is mal debarquement syndrome?"

"We just won't know until we get the test results. But in the meantime, that website will help you understand more about vertigo disorders. I encourage you to check it out."

"I definitely will. Thanks. Also, Dr. Cook told me Valium is the only thing that's been shown to work for mal debarquement. What do you think about that? I really don't want to take benzos, but if they're the only thing—"

"I don't prescribe that stuff. If you want I can prescribe a one-time dose of diazepam to take before the MRI, but that's all I'll do."

Oy, he thinks you're a drug-seeker. "I understand. Is there anything else I might try? I mean it's pretty awful, being constantly on a boat, ha-ha. And again, there's this weird itching, like pinpricks, mostly on my head but kind of everywhere, and my voice is so hoarse, and at night when I'm falling asleep I keep gasping, like my throat is closing up—"

"Have you had any falls?"

"Um, no."

"Your balance is fine? You can walk?"

"Yes."

"Well, I must say your case sounds pretty minor. I have patients in wheelchairs, you know."

Yeah, he thinks you're whining. (Am I whining?) *You shouldn't be whining.*

Dr. Greene said his assistant would call with instructions for scheduling the MRI. I thanked him again and hung up.

———

The Caterpillar and Alice looked at each other for some time in silence: at last the Caterpillar took the hookah out of its mouth, and addressed her in a languid, sleepy voice.

"Who are *you?*" said the Caterpillar.

> ... Alice replied, rather shyly, "I—I hardly know, sir, just at present—at least I know who I was when I got up this morning, but I think I must have been changed several times since then."
>
> "What do you mean by that?" said the Caterpillar sternly. "Explain yourself!"

Among physicians, there are generalists and there are specialists. Generalists treat the patient. Specialists treat the illness. It's important to realize that a specialist is there not to befriend you nor even to notice you, but to evaluate your symptoms, order necessary tests, make a diagnosis, and prescribe a plan of treatment, all of which can be done—indeed, in the specialist's view, *must* be done—with emotional detachment, because he (it's usually, though not always, a he) is addressing an illness, not a person.

> "I can't explain *myself,* I'm afraid, sir," said Alice, "because I'm not myself, you see."
>
> "I don't see," said the Caterpillar.
>
> "I'm afraid I can't put it more clearly," Alice replied very politely, "for I can't understand it myself to begin with, and being so many different sizes in a day is very confusing."
>
> "It isn't," said the Caterpillar.

When you see a specialist, your job as the representative of the illness is to summarize the case as clearly and concisely as possible. You are like a witness in court: you are asked questions, and you answer the questions. You do not ask your own questions, unless invited. You do not meander, waffle, opine, or offer theories. If you do any of these things, the specialist will guide you firmly back on track. This will come across as arrogance, and often it is; more often, however, it is simply the Caterpillar following his process, the process which he believes will lead to correct diagnosis and treatment, and which you are there to assist him with.

> "What size do you want to be?" [the Caterpillar] asked.
>
> "Oh, I'm not particular as to size," Alice hastily replied, "only one doesn't like changing so often, you know."
>
> "I *don't* know," said the Caterpillar.
>
> Alice said nothing; she had never been so much contradicted in all her life before, and she felt that she was losing her temper.

Both Dr. Valentine and Dr. Cook had some Caterpillar qualities, but they lacked the unshakable confidence, penchant for long pauses, and laser-like focus on the illness that define a real Caterpillar. Dr. Greene, now: *He* was a real Caterpillar. Not only was he unshakably confident, given to long pauses, and laser-focused, but he also had that slightly offended air common to his kind: the air of the theoretical physicist intrigued yet repelled by messy experiments, the chief obstetrician captivated yet disgusted by the slime and blood of the birthing womb.

> "Are you content now?" said the Caterpillar.
>
> "Well, I should like to be a *little* larger, sir, if you wouldn't mind," said Alice; "three inches is such a wretched height to be."
>
> "It is a very good height indeed!" said the Caterpillar angrily, rearing itself upright as it spoke (it was exactly three inches high).
>
> "But I'm not used to it!" pleaded poor Alice in a piteous tone. And she thought to herself, "I wish the creatures wouldn't be so easily offended!"

To some Caterpillars, the female body is particularly offensive. Years after the time of this story, I would hear from a friend, a woman in her 70s, who had gone to see Dr. Greene about fluid leaking from her ear. He prescribed an antibiotic. It didn't work. She went back twice more and on the third time, desperate to prove her condition was serious, offered to show him the puppy pad she had used the night before on her pillow to soak up the teaspoon or more of liquid that had seeped out as she slept. Dr. Greene wrinkled his nose in disgust and turned away, scoffing: "It's just an ear infection!" Months later, my friend managed to get a second opinion. Turned out the fluid was cranial fluid, leaking from a skull fracture.

> In a minute or two the Caterpillar took the hookah out of its mouth … Then it got down off the mushroom, and crawled away into the grass, merely remarking as it went, "One side will make you grow taller, and the other side will make you grow shorter."
>
> "One side of *what*? The other side of *what*?" thought Alice to herself.
>
> "Of the mushroom," said the Caterpillar, just as if she had asked it aloud, and in another moment it was out of sight.

I was to meet three more Caterpillars in Madland. Touchy creatures, Caterpillars, with no use for the feelings-before-facts rule; they can be helpful, though, if you know how to handle them.

In mid-August, with the vertigo still constant, the adrenaline surges growing more frequent, and the insomnia worsening, I began a hunt for a saving substance. Somewhere out there, I was certain, there existed a pill, a potion, a mushroom that would calm the storm and, if nothing else, let me sleep. Here are the top-ten hits of my Eat Me Drink Me tour of summer-fall 2020.

#10: Mirtazapine. By means of grovels and snivels, I managed to get an appointment with Dr. Ortega herself: a telemedicine session, which became a regular phone call after we both grew tired of shouting "I can't hear you!" over the static of the video conferencing software. I described my symptoms and hormone adjustments; she encouraged me to keep the hormone regimen as steady as possible, referred me to an endocrinologist (who was booked three months out), and prescribed mirtazapine as a sleep aid. Mirtazapine is an old-time tetracyclic antidepressant, pre-dating the newer SSRIs. At low doses, it acts as a sedative—or so they say. I took it for three nights and found I was more wakeful than ever, so I stopped it.

"But you have to give these things a good try," said Matt.

"If it's making me feel worse, what's the point?" said I.

#9: Neuro-acupuncture. A friend told me about her recent bout of vertigo and the success she'd had with a neuro-acu-puncturist. Round about August 20, I spent an hour in a serene white-plastered feng-shuied office having dainty needles stuck in my head. Dr. Pins was by far the best listener of all the doctors I encountered, giving me a full half hour of transfixed attention as I stood by her desk and recounted my story. She did not suggest supplements or exercise. She did not compare me to her other patients. And she gave every appearance of believing me. But my skepticism rose when I tried to explain my theory of *why* my brain had trapped me on a boat, only to hear her say, as she gently inserted the first needle above my left ear, "Never mind, I don't need to understand the cause of the vertigo in order to treat it." *Say what?*

Her prickly ministrations didn't hurt. They also didn't help.

#8: Alcohol. I'm not much of a drinker. First year in college is the one period in which I drank to excess, a period that came to an end when on the night of my eighteenth birthday I consumed four beers and a sizeable glass of vodka, causing my blood sugar to plummet, which in turn caused a massive panic attack at one in the morning requiring a friend to escort me weeping over to my boyfriend's dorm room and wake him up by pounding on the window, whereupon the boyfriend arose, threw on a jacket, and walked me around campus until I calmed down. I cut way back on the booze after that. But now, increasingly anxious and sleep deprived, and abstinent ever since the No Nap switch had flipped, I thought I'd give alcohol another try. On a warm Friday evening I poured a glass of white wine, settled into the rocking chair, took a sip—and nearly threw up. The No Nap switch, evidently, was also a No Drink switch.

#7: Eyewear. By the last week of August I was spending a portion of each afternoon at the local playground, for swings, like rocking chairs, helped the vertigo. Swaying gently to and fro, I'd shut each eye in turn while reading the Playground Rules sign, 25 feet away. With my right eye, I noticed, the words were not only blurrier but ever-so-slightly doubled. The same was true for street signs. One day I returned home, opened the refrigerator, and was hit in the face by a distortion-field of milk and condiments: *ZUUL!* I made an appointment with my eye doctor. Dr. Lash examined me earnestly, and although she couldn't find a thing wrong with my eyes, she did suggest I discontinue the monovision—that's when your contact lenses correct one eye for distance, the other for reading—and gave me a new glasses prescription. The adjusted contacts and glasses stopped the fridge from Zuuling, but the slight double vision persisted.

#6: Supplements and Thunder Shirts. L-theanine. Holy basil. Turmeric. Magnesium. Progesterone cream. Omega-3 fish oil (lemon flavored, taken by spoon). Vitamin B. Vitamin D. Valerian. By September I had acquired an impressive collection of plastic bottles labeled, "THIS PRODUCT IS

NOT INTENDED TO DIAGNOSE, TREAT, CURE, OR PREVENT ANY DISEASE." A few were suggested by Dr. Ortega or Nurse Practitioner Just-a-Nervous-Girl; most were suggested by Doctor Internet. In an effort to soothe the itchy pain, now flaring in patches on my scalp, face, neck, and torso, I made a trip to a local marijuana dispensary to purchase some cannabidiol cream—non-THC-containing, because *You are not a drug user.* I dosed myself withal, to no avail. Then I recalled how our vet had advised a "thunder shirt" to stop our dog freaking out during bad weather; based on this principle, I bought a weighted blanket, some tight athletic tops, and a vibrating heat pad. Matt, not a fan of weighted blankets or of endless nighttime tossings and turnings, decamped to the Magicouch.

#5: Prednisone. As September progressed, I decided this could not go on. Somehow I managed to get a face-to-face appointment with Dr. Ortega during which I poured out my anguish: the vertigo, I said, was getting worse, not to mention the blurry eyes, the nerve pain, the anxiety, the insomnia. "If only I could sleep standing up," I said, "like a horse!" I was convinced the culprit was the shingles virus attacking my head and ears. "It does *sound* like herpes zoster," said Dr. Ortega. She gave me a week's worth of the oral steroid prednisone and said Dr. Greene could continue it if he agreed. After picking up the pills, I met Matt for lunch at the French bakery across from CVS. He beamed at the news: "Your life is about to change!" As a long-time asthma sufferer, he was a firm believer in prednisone.

He was right: my life was about to change—for the worse. On the prednisone, I alternated between agitation that compelled me to dance maniacally to disco videos and despair that led me, one afternoon, to fall sobbing to my knees begging God to have mercy. At night I lay awake till dawn. After posting on Facebook about the mood swings, I heard from several friends, one of whom described punching a wall in a "prednisone rage."

I called Dr. Greene; his assistant said, "Oh, yeah, some people can't tolerate prednisone." I asked them to taper me off. On the day I stopped it, I slept for nine hours. *Hallelujah,* said Sane Me. *Another mistake, but it's over now. Now maybe you'll get better.* The good news was that the vertigo had abated a tad.

#4: Valacyclovir. Post-prednisone, I started waking up at night feeling I couldn't breathe. Was it Covid? Unlikely, said my friend with an autoimmune disease. Shortness of breath was a symptom of coming off steroids, she said; it would pass. And it did, eventually. What did not pass was the insomnia, which returned in full force along with the adrenaline: awful, buzzing gut-tides of fear that surged out of nowhere, inexorable, irreducible. But I read that these, too, could result from steroid discontinuance. *Ride it out,* said Sane Me. Then, around September 20, I developed a rash on my cheeks. *Just rosacea,* said Sane Me; *still, better get it checked.* When the nurse said yes, it was a shingles rash and I had to take an antiviral right away or risk brain damage, I rushed again to CVS to pick up valacyclovir pills the size of baby carrots. *But it's just rosacea,* whispered Sane Me as I was walking home. I called Dr. Greene's office and asked for advice. They said to hold off on the baby carrots until I could see him.

#3: Acylovir. This time with Dr. Greene, too, I was permitted an in-person visit. I stood outside, behind the yellow line six feet from the door, and thrust out my forehead for the thermometer wielder. The office staff were efficient, cheery. The Caterpillar himself was of slight build, with a head like an egg. He asked when my MRI was happening; I told him October sixth. He allowed me to lower my mask to check the face rash. "Not shingles," he said. "But I have no problem with starting you on an antiviral while we wait for the MRI, just in case this *is* a herpetic infection of some kind. How are you with remembering to take pills?"

"Great," I said.

"Good, then you can do acyclovir. It's five times a day, is the only downside."

"OK by me," I said.

Before leaving, I drew from my purse my bottles of holy basil, turmeric, and L-theanine and asked whether he had an opinion on their value.

"Nope. No opinion. Let me see you out."

#2: Lexapro. Taking the acyclovir five times a day was tedious, but not bad. What was *bad* was my mood, and I'm not talking about I-haven't-had-my-coffee bad or even my-job-sucks bad; more like my-neighbor's-been-running-his-leaf-blower-all-day bad: a physical sense that my nerves were being stretched to the limit, that if I started screaming I might never stop. My ability to focus waned. I stopped writing. When suicidal thoughts began to tiptoe, then to stride around my brain, I called Dr. Ortega; we had a short talk about steroids and acyclovir before I spit it out: "I just want to die!" With evident alarm, she said if I thought I might self-harm I should go to the hospital. (Why, I wondered, is the concern "self-harm"? I didn't want to *harm* myself, I wanted to *fix* myself.) "I just want," I said, "this awful feeling to go away." She prescribed Lexapro, a common SSRI antidepressant.

#1: Ambien. Dr. Ortega warned me that the Lexapro would take a week or two to kick in. I promised patience. But after three nights with a scant two hours of sleep rife with nightmares, including one in which I looked in a mirror to see a psychotic woman's face leering back at me, and another in which Matt stood at the end of the bed grasping and shaking my feet—*Wake up, Bear, wake up!*—I called again and, with a sense of miserable defeat, asked for real, honest-to-god sleeping pills. Dr. Ortega prescribed me 5 milligrams of Ambien, the standard female dose, and suggested I also try melatonin, an over-the-counter sleep hormone. I took half an Ambien the first night, to no effect; tried melatonin the next night, also to no effect; then took a whole Ambien the next nine nights in a row, with the effect that I would be out cold from midnight to three, awaken for an hour, sleep fitfully from four to five, and awaken again to a groggy gray dawn, exhausted but unable to sleep until the next pill at midnight.

It was around this time, I think, that I called the crisis hotline and Hotline Lady told me to box up my scarves and Matt had his first meltdown. "I'm *trying!*" I cried. "You're *not* trying!" he yelled. "You don't stick with anything!" He said this because a day or two earlier I had been to yet another doctor, who had taken me off the Lexapro and put me on yet another drug.

———

"I want you to remember these three words: green, Denver, horse. Repeat them back to me."

"Green, Denver, horse."

"Good. Now, spell 'world' backward."

"D ... um ... d, l ..." Perched on the end of the exam table in Dr. Andersen's office deep in the labyrinth of Mountain Medical Center, I struggled to picture the word *world* backward. *World is w, o, r, l, d, now reverse it, c'mon, it's only one syllable.* "D, l ... um ... r, o, w."

"Now repeat the three words I asked you to remember."

"Green, Denver, horse." (Did I pass? Did I pass?)

Dr. Ortega, upon prescribing the Lexapro, had given me names of a few neurologists. Covid was raging in Santa Fe, making it nearly impossible to get in to see any doctor, let alone a specialist, but when I called Mountain Medical to inquire about Dr. Andersen, they astonished me by saying he had an opening the next day at ten a.m. I booked the appointment.

The facility was fancier than most, with an airy, high-ceilinged lobby guarded by receptionists in germ-safe glass booths and furnished with purple-and-green striped couches that almost matched my purple blazer and green glass earrings. (*Well-groomed!*) Although the buzzing anxiety was now near-constant, I was still able to hide it well enough, and when the ponytailed nurse came to the waiting area to fetch me, I rose, dusted off my purple shoulders, adjusted my mask, and followed her into the labyrinth chatting cordially. The interior was 21st century high-tech, brimming with white, chrome, and beige, like an IKEA.

Nurse Ponytail spent a good fifteen minutes recording my history and symptoms. She also asked me a set of questions about depression. I didn't like having to answer eight of the ten with "yes" or "almost always," but I was determined to be truthful. One question to which I answered "no" was *Do you have a suicide plan?* This, I would later learn, is the main question the pros use in order to gauge depression's severity: if suicidal ideation is a red flag, having a plan is thought to be a much redder flag, a sign you're much closer to doing the deed.[*] The other outlier question was *Do you feel guilty about how your depression is affecting those close to you?* I thought about that for a moment: Did I feel guilty? "No, I can't say I feel *guilty*," I said as Nurse Ponytail typed away, "but I know this whole situation is making things very tough on my husband. Really, I just want to get better." She thanked me and said the doctor would be in shortly.

Dr. Andersen was a big, bodacious Caterpillar. Over six feet, portly, with lank gray hair, he entered the room with a Scandinavian-accented "Good morning!" and dropped himself into the desk chair, the springs of which groaned as he leaned back with knees wide. He clicked his ballpoint pen and held it poised above his clipboard. "Right, Jocelyn, tell me what's going on."

---

[*] Since I went on to make loads and loads of (admittedly half-baked) suicide plans, I don't entirely agree with this perspective, but more on that later.

I was ready. I'd been referring to my notes during Nurse Ponytail's interview; now I consulted them again. "OK, so, since July sixteenth I've had this weird bouncy vertigo, plus nerve pain, insomnia, anxiety, and some other symptoms. This is my second major episode. The vertigo has been diagnosed as this thing called Mal de Débarquement Syndrome, and—"

"Don't look at your notes!"

I jumped. "Sorry, what?"

"Put *away* your notes!" His booming voice pounded my eardrums.

"Oh, sorry, but I need the notes to help me remember. It's hard for me to focus—"

"Put AWAY the notes. Just tell me how it FEELS."

I stared at him as I considered walking out. *Jesus, this guy is an ass. Better humor him.* With an effort, I kept my eyes on his masked face. "OK, well, it feels like I'm on a boat."

"How often do you feel like this?"

"All the time. Except when I'm driving or sitting in a rocking chair."

He scribbled on the chart. "What else?"

"Well, there's this pain, right now it's all over my scalp—"

"What does it feel like?"

"Like a cross between a sunburn and a bruise. Sometimes it's itchy or tingly—"

"How often do you get this pain?"

My eyes dropped to the paper in my lap. I wrenched them back up. "I think this is about the fifth time it's been this bad."

"And what *exactly* does it feel like?"

On we went, back and forth, with him quizzing me about the exact how, when, and where and me trying to answer sans notes. I stressed my sleep problems: "I wake up after a few hours."

"*Why* do you wake up?"

"I don't know."

"You don't *know* why?"

"No, I don't know why." *If we knew why, you numpty, we wouldn't be here!*

I considered saying more about the mood problems and decided not to, figuring that soon he would review what Nurse Ponytail had typed into the computer and see the depression questionnaire. But he never did. He seemed to be inspecting me closely, and after ten minutes of interrogation he put the chart aside, waved his hand at me like a museum tour guide indicating an artwork of negligible interest, and remarked: "You seem relaxed."

I had no idea what to say to that. *We are the very opposite of relaxed, my dear Caterpillar.*

"OK, come up here on the table and let's have a look."

He whizzed through a series of neurological tests: follow finger, squeeze hand, whack knee with rubber mallet, etcetera, wrapping up with the memory challenge: green, Denver, horse. He had me return to the chair and asked if I'd ever had migraine headaches before. "No," I said.

"What about female relatives?" he asked.

"Nope."

"Are you sure? Your mother, sister, an aunt maybe?"

"No, no one." *Yes we know what female relatives are, and none of them has migraines.*

"Hmm. Well, you don't have a brain tumor; tumors don't act like that. This is functional."

"Functional?"

"Not structural. And according to you, you've had this before and you got over it. So you'll probably get over it again."

"Right, but this time it's so much worse." Should I tell him to look at the depression questionnaire? That I think about killing myself? How do I convey suffering without conveying hysteria? "I mean … I feel really, *really* bad. Could it be a virus?"

"No. I believe you have vestibular migraine."

"Oh! Huh. I've read about that, and I did wonder—"

"Yes. I'm going to give you nortriptyline. It's an antidepressant used for migraines, and it will also help you sleep. It's quite sedating. No side effects, except maybe a little blurry vision." He screwed his balled fists into his eyes by way of demonstration: Vision. Blurry.

"What about the Lexapro I'm already on?" *And by the way isn't nortriptyline similar to amitriptyline, which is that stuff the Knave of Hearts said gave him hallucinations?*

"No, Lexapro is good if, like, somebody in your family has died and you're feeling sad. Nortriptyline is better for this."

"Yes, but—"

"Stop the Lexapro. Nortriptyline will be better. 25 milligrams to start. If it's not enough, call me and I'll give you a higher dose. I'll see you again in a month."

The early October sunshine was warm as I crossed the parking lot, clutching the discharge papers with my diagnosis noted in the upper right corner: "Migraine Variants." *Green, Denver, horse. Green, Denver, horse.* I drove to CVS and picked up the new meds.

For the rest of that week, I woke each morning to a sense of Lysol in my veins and an alien spider-beast plastered to my face. Not that I was psychotic, I knew it was the illness, but knowing it was the illness did nothing to mitigate the vibrating, suffocating, sweaty-sick fear. Looking back on it, I suspect it was mostly the Ambien; at the time, however, I blamed Dr. Andersen's nortriptyline. Although I was desperate to rest, lying still, once awake, was becoming impossible. The second morning on the nortriptyline (fourth morning on the Ambien), I staggered into the shower and made the water as hot as I could stand. Water helped. With water running over me, life was almost bearable. But you can't stand in the shower forever.

My mood would improve as the day progressed. I'd made Emily's vacated room my insanity headquarters, having dragged in the big shabby armchair from the living room and rigged up a poster board on top of a folding table as a jigsaw puzzle station. In between my four or five daily walks I'd sit doing puzzles (three hundred pieces of tropical wildlife or holiday snow scenes); needlepointing (two change purses and an eyeglass case, decorated with owls); coloring (a book of flower and bird designs); or working crosswords (*New York Times* Wednesday and Thursday collections). I played folk songs on the piano: Greensleeves, Shenandoah, Oh Where Have You Been, Billy Boy, Billy Boy? After dinner I watched episodes of *Heartland* or *The Great British Baking Show*. But walking and puzzles were the only activities I could sustain for long; anything else and my anxiety, having sat sulking for ten minutes like an attention-deprived toddler, would begin to whine then start tugging on my shirttail—*Mom, Mom, Mom, Mom, Mom*—until I couldn't take it anymore. *Yes, Anxiety, I'm here. I'm here for you, honey.*

Despite all this, Matt continued to insist I was not crazy, that I was in fact getting better. I told him I was ditching the nortriptyline. He said fine, I should go back on the Lexapro. I said the Lexapro hadn't helped, either; at least the Ambien was giving me a few hours of sleep. He said I just had to stick with a regimen, any regimen, and it would work. He assigned me chores to do around the house and garden: "If you keep busy you'll feel better." At his bidding I swept the front porch, cleaned the outdoor light fixtures, washed the windows, watered the shrubs, weeded the driveway. I walked four or five miles each day. I dropped five pounds, then ten.

On October sixth, we drove to get my MRI. After my first visit with Dr. Greene I had investigated MRI options in Santa Fe and found to my dismay that there were no open or wide-bore machines, only the slide-in vampire tubes, whereupon I googled farther afield and discovered a place in Albuquerque called Southwest Upright MRI. Their website showed a smiling young woman seated in a sort of space pod; the sides of the pod touched her shoulders, but the front was open, and they said you could watch TV (CHOOSE FROM 150 CHANNELS!) during your scan. Upright space pod sounded much better than vampire tube. When I called them they were very nice and said yes, they took Blue Cross Blue Shield. In the days leading up to the event I practiced sitting still in a chair for as long as possible, timing myself and building to 20 minutes, which I knew wasn't long enough—MRIs take 30 to 45 minutes—but I figured practice of any length could only help. I also pondered which TV channel to select.

I was dismayed afresh, upon our arrival, to see that Southwest Upright MRI presented not as a gleaming medical facility but as a slightly grimy strip-mall storefront. ALL SHOES HALF PRICE shouted a banner in the window next door. *Whatever. It's upright. You wanted upright. Upright is better.* We entered a waiting room decorated in 1990s Florida Dentist Office and filled out forms for a businesslike woman behind a Plexiglas barrier. I said I wanted my husband to be in the room with me.

"Due to Covid, only the patient is allowed in the scan room." She gave me a look as if to say: *Your move.*

Having studied their website, I was prepared. "It's medically necessary."

"No problem." She pushed a few more forms through the slot. "Sign here, and here."

After a short wait we were taken back to a changing cubicle. I was handed more forms and swore that I did not have a hip implant, an IUD, a pacemaker, or a microchip. I swore I was not allergic to the contrast dye they would inject for the second half of the scan. I swore I would drink lots of water afterward. I took off everything from the waist up and wrapped a voluminous cotton gown around my torso, then two young female techs came and led us to the scan room, where I was given a choice of seat cushions, waffled or non (I chose non), and assisted into the space pod. One of the techs placed a chair for Matt a few feet in front of me to my right. She indicated the TV on the wall. "What do you want to watch?" she asked.

"Do you have music channels?"

"No."

"How about HGTV," Matt said. "You like HGTV."

"Fine," I said.

The tech clicked the remote to summon the handsome faces of the Property Brothers, who were presiding over a home-make-over team challenge. Meanwhile the other tech gave me a pair of yellow foam earplugs to insert, lowered a plastic football helmet over my head, and stuffed pillows on either side of my neck. "Here we go," she said. She pressed a button, causing the sides of the pod to close in tight as the chair levitated three feet up, slid four feet aft, and tilted backward at a 45-degree angle, all with a smooth mechanical whir, like a tray sliding into an Easy Bake Oven.

"Comfy? Now remember, stay absolutely still whenever you hear the really loud banging noises." Both techs left the room.

You know … upright may not be better.

————

I made it through, though I couldn't have told you a single thing about the home makeovers or which Property Brother won the challenge. The machine's noise was like a jackhammer, and I focused all my dwindling store of willpower on breathing and not moving, suspended up there in my jackhammer space-pod Easy Bake Oven. The first part took 35 minutes, after which they lowered the chair, injected the contrast dye into my wrist, and set me to bake for another 15 minutes. Matt turned and waved at me every so often; I responded with a thumbs-up.

On the drive home, he said in his buck-you-up voice, "Now that that's over, I expect dramatic improvement!" I was just relieved to be done.

I called Dr. Greene's office the next day to inquire about my results. His assistant called back: "Good news, nothing abnormal." No tumor, no cyst, no signs of multiple sclerosis. But Matt's expectations for dramatic improvement were not met, for I had pinned my hopes on getting an explanation, no matter how dire, for what was happening to me. Cancer or MS would have at least provided a clear treatment path to follow; with this "good news," the path was as obscure as ever.

I made a follow-up appointment with Dr. Greene and at the same time decided to shift my focus to finding some type of psychiatric care. Way back in August, aware that I probably needed help coping emotionally with the resurgent vertigo, I had embarked on a search for a therapist; after running into dead end after dead end (because Covid), I messaged a psychologist friend to ask for a referral to someone, anyone, even if they didn't take insurance. My friend came through with a referral to Denise, a Jungian therapist, with whom I completed one session then ditched in order to set out on the Eat Me Drink Me tour, which had seemed the right idea at the time. At the end of September, the tour having flopped, I called Therapist Denise and begged her to take me back. She very kindly did. I asked her for names of psychiatrists—by this point I wanted someone who could prescribe meds, not just offer counsel—and she recommended three, two of whom I called only to be told they weren't taking new patients. The third one, however, had space on his roster.

Alas, it turned out that this doctor's assistant was renowned in the local community for her, how shall I say?—lack of concern for the patient experience. (Months later, Therapist Denise would snort, "Oh yeah, that woman is a bitch and a half.") Desperate, I pressed forward anyway and booked two in-person appointments, the first for picking up intake forms and the second for dropping off intake forms, but the assistant's bored hostility, which she did not trouble to hide, left me more drained and dejected than ever. Moreover, the doctor himself had no openings until mid-December.

I could feel body and spirit wading deeper into the mire, the watery muck oozing up to my ankles ... to my knees ... soon it would be up to my thighs. The more I struggled, the lower I sank. There had to be someone, somewhere, who would throw me a line.

I typed "mental health residential facility" into the Google search bar and hit Enter.

PART II

LOOKING-GLASS HOUSE

CHAPTER 5

ALL THE RUNNING
YOU CAN DO

~~~~~~~~~~~~~~~~~~~~~~

The True Healing Center is (or was; it has since closed) a short drive from Santa Fe out the Old Las Vegas Highway. You turn right half a mile past Harry's Roadhouse, dip under the I-25 overpass, travel another twisty quarter mile through the standard high-desert landscape of juniper trees and piñons, yellow-brown grass and sage brush, then make a left at the sign. It's an easy trip from a logistical standpoint; from an emotional standpoint, not so much.

The sun was just beginning its descent from the zenith as Matt and I rolled up to the site on Tuesday, October thirteenth, for my scheduled admission. There was a driveway leading to a small parking lot, but nothing indicating reception, so we continued on for fifty yards—a prickly wooded slope on our right, a coyote fence on our left—until we were stopped by a black metal gate pulled halfway across a gap between two pillars.

"This isn't it," Matt said.

"Must be back there," I said, all my energy focused on not-disintegrating.

He swung the Jeep around and drove back to the parking lot. There were a few other cars there; no people. He pulled in and shut off the engine. An immense, dry quiet greeted us.

Since making these arrangements three days ago, I'd been picturing the True Healing Center as something like a certain four-star resort in Scottsdale, Arizona, where I'd once attended an industry conference: cream-colored stucco buildings, raked gravel footpaths, guests in business casual roaming here and there, flowering cacti, maybe a koi pond. These picturings were based on the center's website plus my natural visualization ability, which approximates that of a blind mole rat. *When are you going to learn that nothing is ever, ever as you imagine it?* Sane Me remarked as we got out of the Jeep and looked around at the unassuming facility, more campers' motel than four-star resort. I could see half a dozen low, adobe-style structures mixed with aluminum-sided trailers in a space the size of a large playground. A couple of asphalt walkways snaked through hard-packed dirt dotted with shrubs and weeds. Down one path in the near distance, a gazebo of plywood kept the sun off the heads of four or five smokers. Around the horizon, the Sangre de Cristo foothills slumped in fuzzy folds, uncaring.

Last week I had asked the intake coordinator about the center's demographics. I had a vague sense that "true healing" really meant "drug rehab," and I didn't want to be the one crazy old lady amid a couple dozen tattooed twenty-somethings whose parents had packed them off to detox where they couldn't embarrass said parents in front of their friends. Later I would find that my tattooed twenty-something roommate was my favorite person in the joint; still, I was relieved when the intake coordinator said the center's "clients" were typically a mix of old and young, that older folks predominated at the moment, and that many of them suffered from anxiety, depression, and other mental illnesses instead of, or alongside of, substance abuse. She had spoken, she said, with the center's chief psychiatrist, who had said yes, they could help me, and yes, I should come. My expected stay: one month.

I'd planned to check in after lunch, which I figured would give me time to go in the morning to Santa Fe's early voting location and cast my ballot; necessary, since I would be shut away (healing, presumably) on Election Day itself. I'd resolved to vote even if I had to crawl downtown on hands and knees and wait forever. In fact I walked, and the wait at the county building was about an hour. As I stood with several hundred of my fellow citizens in the line circling the courtyard, all of us advancing, inchworm-like, from one social-distance footprint sticker to the next, I observed that although the anxiety and itching remained severe, the vertigo wasn't too bad. Surely I'd survive without a rocking chair for a month. Wouldn't I?

Mad Me: Please don't make me go!

Sane Me: *You will go.*

We had arrived, Matt and I, a little before my one-thirty check-in time. We still couldn't see a sign for reception, and there was no one around to ask. Two small buildings flanked the parking area; we approached one, climbed a flight of wooden steps, and cupped our hands to peer through a window into a darkish room with stainless steel refrigerators, coffee urns, and a long table. "Cafeteria," Matt said. The pandemic plus my shot nerves summoned up a scenario (Maybe they're all *dead*) wherein everyone had succumbed to a contagious disease, leaving behind a ghost town—but no, there were the smokers in the gazebo. We crossed the parking lot to the other building. This one had a blue door topped by a sign that said *Beginnings*; looking through the glass pane we could see a space with a couple of chairs, a stack of cardboard boxes, and what looked like a reception desk. Matt tried the handle: locked. He knocked: no response. For a minute we stood there at a loss, staring through the glass as the immense, dry quiet persisted. Finally a man in a maintenance uniform came around a corner inside, exited, and held the door for us, not saying a word. We thanked him and went on through.

In a looking-glass house, you keep expecting to move forward only to find yourself moving backward or, at any rate, not in the direction you'd hoped. Said the Red Queen to Alice: *Here, it takes all the running you can do to keep in the same place!* This sense of flailing non-progress persisted through my five-night stay at the True Healing Center—yes, only five nights; I checked in on Tuesday, checked out on Sunday, and because they are not the Hotel California, they let me leave. My first 24 hours there unfolded as follows.

————

Late afternoon. I had assumed there'd be many administrative hoops to jump, so I wasn't too fazed by the six-inch stack of forms plus four-thousand-dollar copay, the urine test, nurse exam, handover of prescription meds, and swab up nose for Covid. I had also assumed, however, that once those hoops were cleared I would be seen by a psychiatrist. This did not happen. Instead, at three-thirty I was sent from the exam room back to the reception area "to wait for the client tech who'll check you into your cabin." Piled by a chair was my overlarge collection of luggage: roller bag, backpack, tote bag, purse, weighted blanket, coat, and Elephant. (Well, it was supposed to be for a month!) I took a seat beside the pile with hands shaking, eyes welling. I was alone: after the forms, Matt had been told to go. I clung to him as we said goodbye, sensing his worry mixed with some relief at having the mad wife off his plate.

On check-in I had warmed to the young receptionist, who'd complimented my necklace in a kind and friendly way. I now asked her when I'd be seeing a doctor. "Oh, you'd like to see the doctors?" she said, as if this were a special request. "I'll see if I can get you in this evening."

Get me in? I thought I *was* in. This was not promising. But after a while she leaned across the desk to say I had an appointment with "the doctors" at 7:30 p.m. So that was all right. I took out a crossword book and blinked back the tears, resolving to trust the process, to trust that this was a good place. I managed to interact normally enough with a strapping blond man in navy-blue polo shirt and matching facemask who came by and introduced himself as the CEO of True Healing, repeating somewhat inanely, "We're glad you're here! We're glad you're here!" I supposed the greeting was meant as a buoyant counterpoint to the non-gladness felt, no doubt, by the majority of new—patients? guests? residents? No, the term was *clients*. I was a *client*.

At four o'clock, my escort showed up. "Number 7, thanks, Lorena!" said Kind Friendly Receptionist. Client Tech Lorena was short and stocky, her manner businesslike. She hoisted my backpack and roller bag, leaving tote bag, purse, weighted blanket, coat, and Elephant to me, and led the way to a row of cabins that curved along one side of a flagstone yard dotted with concrete benches and juniper trees. The building containing Numbers 7 and 8 was at the end of the row. It looked all right from the outside, and I was just telling myself we were getting somewhere at last when CT Lorena unlocked the door to reveal ...

Oh, hell no.

The room had three beds. One had clearly been occupied a short while ago; it lay unmade, a sticky detritus of paper cups, damp towels, food wrappers, used tissues, and other trash strewn about. The other two beds had no linens, no pillows, just a stained coverlet pulled up over the mattress. One had a side table with a lamp: ripped shade, no lightbulb. The double-socket wall bracket held a single bulb, which illuminated when Lorena flipped the switch but served to reduce the gloom no better than the dirty window with its broken, sagging blind. Dust coated every surface. Crumbs littered the floor. The stench of mildew made my eyes sting.

I had no idea how to react. Was this a mistake? Was this just how things were in a healing center? But I'm a *client*, I thought. You shouldn't treat clients like this. Also, the photos on your website are very misleading.

CT Lorena glanced around with a frown. "Huh. Looks like it hasn't been cleaned."

This is a bad place, I thought.

"I'll tell them to get Housekeeping in here. Which bed do you want?"

"Um, I guess this one." I pointed at the one with the lamp. Maybe they could get me a lightbulb. And a pillow. And some sheets.

"Fine. So, now I need to do your inventory. Basically you need to take everything out of your bags, and I write it down." She sat down at the desk, clipboard at the ready. "I have to write down every single thing. Start wherever you want."

Mad Me: Wait, what? No!! I am a client, not a prisoner! I hate you, CT Lorena!

Sane Me: *Oh my god, calm down. They have to check for drugs. Just do as she says.*

I swung my roller bag atop a dresser, unzipped it, and began to unpack, showing and naming each item of clothing before placing it in a drawer. "One sweatshirt." She wrote it down. "One pair jeans." She wrote it down. "Nine, ten pairs of under-pants. Pajamas. One sweater ..."

I really thought I had packed judiciously, but as the heap grew I had a momentary vision of my clothes overflowing the dresser, filling the room and spilling out the door. I finished the roller bag and asked Lorena if I should do the backpack next. "Up to you," she shrugged. The backpack held a gallon-sized bag-gie of toiletries, which she inspected to be sure none contained alcohol ("A lot of moisturizers do"), along with books—for reading, crosswords, coloring—none of which gave her pause, but when I pulled out a small blue pencil sharpener: "Let me see that." She examined it closely. "Yeah, you can't have this. It's got a razor blade. It needs to be locked up at the nurses' station. You can sign it out for ten minutes a day."

"Seriously?"

"Yes. No sharps allowed in the rooms."

Her mention of *sharps* cast the situation in a new and ominous light. I had in my tote bag a pair of scissors and my needlepoint kit—which included, obviously, needles, though they were pretty blunt needles—and in my purse a small makeup bag that contained a nail clipper. It became suddenly very apparent that these items were contraband, and very important that I *not* be stripped of needlepoint or nail clipper. *Give her the scissors,* said Sane Me, moving smoothly into the role of criminal mastermind. *That'll demonstrate transparency; then she might overlook the other illegal stuff.*

Having handed over the scissors and emptied the backpack, I gestured casually to my blanket and Elephant as if to say, "That's all," whereupon Lorena stood up—but her eye fell on the tote bag and purse. "Did we do those?" she asked.

"Oh! I guess not." *Damn.*

"OK, what's in those." She re-poised the clipboard with an air of impatience.

I knelt down with my back to her and pulled items from the tote, tossing them onto the bed: "One crossword book ... one box of colored pencils ... one hairbrush ..." The needlepoint kit was flat, unobtrusive. I left it deep in the tote and moved on to the purse. "Water bottle ... house keys ... reading glasses ... wallet ..." Next was the makeup bag (*Be cool!*), but at the wallet's appearance Lorena seemed to lose interest in the inventory and segued into an explanation of how valuables were stored. Awash with relief at my successful concealment of needlepoint and nail clipper, I told her she could take and lock up my wallet.

"I don't have to," she said, suddenly conciliatory. "It's for your own peace of mind."

But I said yes, take it, which set in motion a chain of increasingly tense ruminations as Lorena toured me briskly around the facility, reciting the house rules and the purposes of various buildings, none of which I absorbed because I was obsessing about my wallet's absence. When she dropped me off back at Number 7, I stood in the middle of the floor intoning, "God help me. God help me," then hurried over to Reception to grip the edge of the desk while informing Kind Friendly Receptionist that I wanted my wallet back and wanted it now.

Kind Friendly said of course, she understood. She called Lorena's cell phone as I waited, swaying and sniffling. Her side of the dialogue went something like this:

"Hi, Lorena. I have Jocelyn here. She's just told me she wants to keep her wallet ... Yes, I know ... Mm hmm ... Well, she's had a change of heart ... OK, Lorena, thank you so much."

As for Lorena's side, I imagine it boiled down to: "For fuck's sake. *Clients!*"

―――――――

Early evening. I was required to stay in quarantine until my Covid test came back clear. "Friday at the earliest," Lorena had said. Quarantined newbies could not, in theory, enter the cafeteria or join group activities, though it turned out in practice nobody barred us from the cafeteria outside of formal mealtimes, nor did anyone prevent or even discourage us from participating in group activities as long as we didn't sit too close. Our meals were brought to us on trays. And (thank heaven) we got to keep our phones until such time as we "joined the community."

I met Roberto, head of Maintenance, when he came by Number 7 to drop off the dinner menu. Bearded and jovial, he sticks in my memory as an exemplar of the truth that in unhappy situations nothing beats humanity—and by "humanity" I mean "treating someone like a fellow human being." After introducing himself and handing me the menu, he glanced around and said with a grimace, "Wow, this place is a mess. We're going to have to move you."

"Oh! Thank you!"

"Sorry 'bout that. We're short-staffed because of Covid. I'll just need to get the other room sanitized and then I'll help you move your stuff."

"No problem!" I wanted to hug him.

After I'd circled a few food items—chicken and cheese sandwich, side salad with ranch dressing, milk to drink—he asked if I'd been shown around. "Yes," I said. "Well, kind of."

"Here, lemme give you the tour." He proceeded to take me on his version, which I recall as being much more informative and relaxed than Lorena's, though admittedly I was in a better frame of mind now, having made four circuits of the facility's walking path and returned to the room to find my wallet sitting on the desk. I put wallet in purse and took purse with me as we strolled around, Roberto providing the inside scoop on everything from laundry to computer time to snagging covert snacks from the kitchen. He indicated the perimeter of the property: "Make sure you don't go beyond it, or they'll think you're eloping." The word made me think of Vegas weddings. "If you elope, we have to call the sheriff. It's a whole thing. Also, see that road? The guy who lives down there has some mean dogs." I imagined myself going Butch and Sundance, racing over the hills with sheriff's posse and mean dogs in ferocious pursuit. Then I remembered it would be an easy walk to Harry's Roadhouse where I could get an Uber, or actually, since I still had my phone, I could get the Uber to come right here. As if reading my mind, Roberto said, "This is why we lock up your luggage, see." Right, right ... Lorena had taken my roller bag. I still had my backpack and purse, though ... and my wallet ... then again, they had my meds. I couldn't elope without my meds. *Jesus Christ, you are not going to elope!*

Roberto brought my dinner tray at six p.m. and suggested I sit outside to eat, on a bench by the flagstone circle. "Then I'll help you move your stuff into Number 1," he said.

The whole place still seemed strangely empty, but as I wiped my hands of chicken grease in preparation for tackling the ranch dressing packet, two women came strolling along the walkway. They approached me, smiling.

"Hi!" said the shorter, perkier one with the chubby face. "I'm Daphne, and this is my roommate, Delia! Are you new? Did you just arrive?"

"Um, hi." *Pull it together.* "Yes, hello! I got here this afternoon. I'm Jocelyn."

"Welcome, Jocelyn! It's awful being new! Don't worry, it gets better once you're out of quarantine! This is a good place! We've been here three weeks! What room are you in?"

"I was in Number 7, but I guess they're moving me to Number 1."

Delia, the taller, slimmer one with the pointy face, nodded graciously and said nothing.

"Oh good, you'll be right near us!" Daphne chirped. "Well, it's nice to meet you! We have to go to dinner! Feel free to ask me about anything! Glad you're here! Bye now!"

"See you later! Thanks!" I waved gaily at them as they left, then turned back to do battle with the dressing packet. I was grateful to have been welcomed by two old hands; at the same time, Daphne's in-your-face cheeriness combined with Delia's superior silence creeped me out a little. I was reminded of orientation week at boarding school, tenth grade, when I'd been constantly on the verge of tears and amazed at how nonchalant all the other kids seemed.

But when at 6:45 I lugged my backpack, tote bag, purse, and blanket up the walkway to Number 1, Roberto leading the way with a plastic laundry hamper full of my clothes and books, and the door opened onto a clean oak floor, three beds neatly made with olive-green quilts, a lamp on each bedside table, armchair, armoire, two desks under the window—gratitude swamped every other emotion. Rustic? Sure. And compared with Number 7, it might as well have been the Ritz. "This is better, huh?" laughed Roberto.

Again I suppressed the urge to hug him. "*Much* better!"

He left me to my second round of unpacking, and as I placed Elephant on the bed next to the window, I thought: Maybe I did the right thing. Maybe this really is a good place.

————

After dinner. Each building on the campus had a name: Unity, Vision, Wellness, Harmony, Serenity … *Where's Batshittery? ha-ha.* Unity, a high-mounted double-wide trailer, housed the meds dispensary, nurses' station, doctors' offices, and contraband drawers. After Roberto's tour I'd gone there for my afternoon dose of acyclovir and had encountered two other residents. One was a statuesque middle-aged woman with glasses, who introduced herself as Janet; like Daphne, she exuded top notes of cheer with undertones of mania and was, she said, checking out her credit card. (I peeked at my wallet in my purse.) The other was a teenage girl, thin, dark-haired, in denim shorts. She sat with hands between knees, her body trembling, fawnlike, as she talked quietly with Janet. A ladder of cut marks scored each of her pale thighs.

Down in my gut, splinters of shock, pity, and revulsion merged into a jagged sphere and careened around like a pinball.

Statuesque Janet waved me ahead of her at the counter, and I asked for my meds. "No," said the staffer on duty, "you need to go around back. Covid rules. You wait outside and we take one at a time." I went out and around the trailer to find a few folks waiting by plywood stairs to the back door. Under a pine tree, a couple of benches and an Adirondack chair provided seating.

The sky was sheer blue, the air brisk. It took about five minutes for each person to get in and out, a fifteen-minute wait in
total, which didn't seem bad; I would discover, however, that
the pre-bedtime rush was quite another thing, and on nights
to come I would join a slew of other inmates, all freezing our
asses off beneath the spectacular New Mexico stars as we chatted,
smoked, or stared for an hour or more until we were summoned
to the magic window through which a lone, harried nurse would,
with all due process and paperwork, dispense our pills.

Unity's front entrance was mainly for medical visits. At
7:28 p.m., I presented myself again at the desk and tried to look
legitimate. The three staffers kept their eyes on their computers.
"Hello," I said to the air. No response. "Hello! I have an appointment with the doctors." A frown was directed my way, a fore-
stalling hand raised. I stepped back and waited. *Hello! My name
is Inigo Montoya. You killed my father. Prepare to die.* A white
board on the wall displayed tomorrow's therapist appointments;
I saw my name down for 1:30 with "Natalie."

At length I was called beyond the counter and presented to
the folks in charge: a nurse practitioner whose name I promptly
forgot and, *hallelujah*, "our attending psychiatrist, Dr. Anna
Funar." The doctor was 40ish, jeans, light brown hair in a ponytail, with a Romanian accent and a beaming benevolence that
came across as professional yet genuine. Her warm manner
emboldened me to say, "Hi, Anna!" (I immediately regretted it
and called her "Dr. Funar" forevermore.) She ushered me into
her cramped office, apologized for the mess, cleared a chair of a
stack of journals, and invited me to sit. She offered me a cup of
water, which I accepted. Then she sat down across from me and,
with her Cheshire Cat smile waxing and waning but never quite
disappearing, listened to my story.

Though my anxiety kept up its usual keening whine throughout the interview—*Mom, Mom, Mom, Mom, Mom*—and I was
trembling almost as badly as the fawn girl with the cut marks,

Dr. Funar's gentle attention steadied me. I told her about the vertigo, the insomnia, the anxiety, the skin pain, the suicidal ideation. I told her about all the meds I'd tried and how the Lexapro had seemed to make things worse, though I'd only been on it for three days so to be fair I didn't really know. I asked her whether I might try Celexa—for the terribly scientific reason that my friend Susan's husband had taken it—to which she replied, "No, I think Zoloft is best in your case," and something about the way she said it, the quickness combined with assurance, made me think that here, at long last, was someone who knew what to do. I said the controlled-release Ambien was giving me three, maybe four hours of sleep. Since it was doing some good, she said, I should try the higher dose, the one usually reserved for men, because "restoring sleep comes first." *It does, it does.* She asked me about substance abuse, childhood abuse, domestic violence, sexual assault; I wondered what percentage of the center's clients had a history of all four, unlike me, who had none, and wondered again what my excuse was for taking up everyone's time. I asked her about benzodiazepines; she said yes, she thought I'd be helped by clonazepam, brand name Klonopin, and when I expressed concern about it being addictive she said, "Well, but if you need it, you need it. If you break your leg, you need crutches."

My chin lifted at the insight. "If you break your leg, you need crutches," I repeated. "And if you break your brain ..."

"You need crutches for your brain," she laughed. "That's right."

"Wow. That makes so much sense."

She said she'd prescribe me Zoloft—or rather its generic equivalent, sertraline—at 25 milligrams, but I should break the pills in half to start, since I was clearly sensitive to medication. Clonazepam at 0.5 milligrams, which I should also break in half and take as needed. Ambien CR, 12.5 milligrams, the man-sized dose. And the hormones and acyclovir could stay as they were.

I wrote it all down in the slim brown notebook they'd given me at check-in. "The only thing to be careful about," she warned, "is to leave at least two hours between the clonazepam and the Ambien, because Ambien is a benzo derivative, so you don't want to combine them."

"I understand. Thank you" (for treating me like an intelligent person).

As our meeting concluded, she explained that she worked at another clinic during the day, arriving here in late afternoon, which was why appointments were always in the evening. She said I could make another appointment whenever I felt the need. And she showed me the diagnoses she'd written on my chart: Generalized anxiety disorder. Panic disorder. Depression.

Well, fine, said Sane Me as I exited the office. *We still don't know what's causing any of it, but at least somebody gets that our brain needs crutches.*

––––––––

Late evening. "Hi, I'm Jocelyn."

"Hi, Jocelyn!" the circle intoned.

I was sitting on a floor pillow, back to the wall, in the shiplapped meeting room of Vision, the building next door to Unity. Some two dozen other clients perched on folding chairs and windowsills or sat cross-legged on the floor like me, our fleece pullovers zipped tight against the dry, wood-scented cold; maybe fifteen women, eight men, a wide variety of ages, shades, and sizes. On the couch at the top of the circle sat Cameron and Jack.

I'd met these two on my way to this evening wrap-up session; they had greeted me with warmth (and without, thankfully, the frantic vibes of Perky Daphne and Statuesque Janet) and complimented my courage in going to a group activity my first night. "Gosh, you're brave," said Jack. "My first few days, I hid in my room." Yeah, I'd prefer to be hiding, too, I thought, but as my mother used to say: *Take everything that's going.*

Cameron and Jack looked to be in their late twenties. Cameron was tall, ash blonde, soccer-girl pretty; Jack was short, brown-eyed, nerdily handsome. I pegged them as the cool kids, the popular, outgoing pair united in their strategy to be last voted off the island, and my assessment was confirmed when they entered the Vision meeting room at 8:35 to take their seats on the couch, which had been left empty for them, and Cameron said, "OK, let's get started." She was, evidently, the appointed peer leader of the gathering. All the CT in attendance did was to take people's temperatures as they arrived, then join the circle for Sharing.

Ah, Sharing, the prime directive of the therapeutic universe. Sharing is Caring. Sharing is the Way. At this evening circle, each person was supposed to share their daily intention (which they had shared at the morning circle), then share how they'd done with that intention, and then, if they wanted, share something for which they were grateful. I was sitting at the ring's midpoint, so I had examples to follow; mostly the gratitude was for loved ones—children, siblings, partners—with whom the person was in contact (phone privileges were three times a week for 30 minutes), and the intentions were about either "staying positive" or "making progress on one of my projects." I didn't know what a "project" was. There seemed to be a required set of them about which I hadn't yet been informed, and this realization caused my standard anxiety dream, the one where I've forgotten to go to class all semester and the paper is due tomorrow, to swim up from the depths of my subconscious and tweak my toes, but Sane Me kicked it roughly back down to the seabed: *Never mind about projects, it's your first night for god's sake.*

One by one the inmates shared. "Hi, I'm Teresa." "Hi, I'm Bill." "Hi, I'm Cody." "Hi, I'm Lark." Roommates Daphne and Delia were there, sitting side by side. Statuesque Janet was there. The fawn girl was not there; this circle consisted solely of adults who were, as far as I could tell, quite high functioning, although

93

I could sense a miasma of stress and pain hanging over us like stale cigarette smoke. Any remotely positive statement—even "I accomplished nothing on my project today"—was greeted with finger snaps. *All have won, and all must have prizes, said the Dodo.* After each person's contribution, the group chorused: "We support you!"

I was feeling confident (or what passed for confident), having in my corporate-training life participated in and presided over many similar rounds. When it came my turn:

"Hi, I'm Jocelyn."

"Hiiii, Jocelyn!"

"It's my first night here," [finger snaps, murmurs of welcome] "so I didn't set any goals, ha-ha" [finger snaps]. "But I'm really grateful to be here and looking forward to meeting you all. I also just want to say I'm grateful for my daughter. I got to talk with her earlier this evening. She lives in Austin, she's great, and I'm so happy to have her in my life." [finger snaps] "Thanks."

"We support yooou!"

Nailed it.

Leader Cameron was the last to speak. She began as she would begin every night—"My intention for the day was to tell negative thoughts to fuck off"—and went on to express gratitude for I forget what. Then we all got to our feet and shuffled in to form a tighter circle, wherein we recited the Serenity Prayer: "God grant me the serenity to accept the things I cannot change, the courage to change the things I can, and the wisdom to know the difference." Next came a loud chant, "Keep coming back! It works if you work it!" followed by a little dance, forward-kick-forward-kick-turn-around-backward-kick, after which the group broke up and dispersed.

I never mastered the little dance or grasped its meaning. Maybe someday, someone will clue me in.

Nighttime. The first major setback was when they mislaid the Ambien.

I'd borne the ass-freezing, 60-minute wait with the crowd behind Unity secure in the belief that although the meds Dr. Funar had ordered wouldn't arrive until tomorrow, the meds I'd brought with me would be there and available. But when it came my turn at the magic window, my Ambien had gone missing. Each client's prescriptions were kept in a gallon-sized baggie in a giant filing cabinet in the meds room, alphabetized by last name. The nurse easily located my progesterone and acyclovir; controlled substances, however, were kept in separate, locked drawers, and for some reason the Ambien bottle wasn't there with the other D's. (It transpired next day that the baggie had been misfiled.) They often had backup supplies of common drugs, the nurse said, but gosh, sorry, all out of Ambien.

There was clearly nothing I could do, so I swallowed my orange progesterone Skittle and blue-striped acyclovir capsule—you had to take your meds under the nurse's eye—and left.

Back at Number 1, Sane Me delivered another pep talk about trusting the process. I was alone in the cabin and glad of that; at least I didn't have to cope with a roommate. I took a shower, got into my pajamas, and settled myself in the armchair with my coloring book and pencils. Roberto stopped by to see how I was; I thanked him again for the extra pillows he'd scrounged for me after I'd explained about the vertigo. "Oh yeah, my wife has that," he'd said. Next to pop in was the young CT who had been at the wrap-up circle: her name was Pat, and she explained she was on duty that night and would be checking on me every two hours.

"Every two hours? Really?"

"Yes," she said with a shrug. "It's policy. We try to be super quiet. I hope the flashlight doesn't wake you."

"Oh, no worries." *It won't wake us, babe, because we'll be awake.*

After she left I turned down the room's thermostat and got into bed, where I did a crossword and waited for the vertigo waves to subside. The anxiety was, as usual, at its lowest ebb for the day. The pressure of the weighted blanket was pleasant, and the heat worked fine. All in all things could be worse, I thought, as I turned off the light and curled up on my left side with head propped on three pillows, Elephant tucked beneath my chin.

The night crept by.

And by.

And by.

I made sure to keep my eyes closed every time the door creaked open and the flashlight beam fell on my face. I didn't want CT Pat to think I wasn't trying.

As the birds in the piñons outside the window began to trill, I drifted off for, twenty minutes? Thirty? I know I did fall asleep, because I had a dream about eloping from the healing center and hitching a ride down a dark, lonely road in a white van driven by Roberto only to end up at some sort of party house where I wandered from room to room asking partygoers if they knew the way home (*but answer came there none*). When I awoke, I looked at the bedside clock: five-fifteen. I lay watching the air in the room lighten from charcoal to dishwater gray, feeling the pitiless fear-tide rising, rising, over the riverbank … up the levee … higher, higher, until, unable any longer to keep my finger in the dike, I sat up and commenced picking frantically, painfully, at the dry skin on my heels. *Just like the fawn girl's cutting*, said Sane Me. *I know, the body pain distracts you from the mind pain. Good thing no one sees the soles of your feet, right?*

At six a.m., CT Pat entered and found me like that. "You doing OK? Did you sleep at *all?*" she asked in a voice of sympathy, switching off the flashlight.

"Not really." I clasped my hands atop the blanket. "Maybe half an hour."

"Would you like anything? Some tea?"

"OK ... yes, please. Do you have peppermint?"

"Absolutely. Peppermint tea, coming up."

The tea helped a little. I ate a third of a protein bar from the supplies in my tote bag. When the clock said 6:30, I got up and took another shower.

I hadn't expected to get much shuteye without the Ambien, but sheesh—half an hour? Standing under the hot spray, I thought about all the insomnia-conquering advice I'd read and the methods I'd tried in recent months: the relaxation techniques, the sleep hygiene practices, the lullabies-for-baby YouTube videos—8 HOURS, NO ADS—the supplements, the teas, the apps where Meryl Streep reads you bedtime stories. Therapist Denise had confessed she herself was "a bad sleeper" and suggested I try audiobooks: "They're so soothing. All you have to do is press a button on your phone." In online forums I'd eavesdropped on scores of insomniacs sharing their woes and tips, many of whom talked about how their anxiety was linked to sleep. But I hadn't found anyone, in person or online, who seemed to understand my particular type of sleep anxiety.

You see, I wasn't scared of going to sleep. I was scared of waking up.

Because waking up, I knew, is when I would face the punishment for having slept. My reptilian brain, now set to permanent red alert, had appointed itself my security detail: its job was to protect me from the storm about to hit, the bombs about to drop. If I slept, how could it protect me? If I slept, who could tell what disasters might befall me unaware? Our brain is designed to keep us alive, not to keep us happy, and my brain (or a deep, atavistic part of it) had decided the only way to keep me alive was to keep me awake. So, if I did fall asleep—thanks to sheer exhaustion or strong drugs, either of which might silence the air raid siren for a few hours—if I *did* fall asleep, Security Brain was going to make me pay. At the earliest sign of consciousness, she would crank up the siren to eleven. She would send in the whip-wielding demon to give me fifty lashes, laid without mercy atop the oozing stripes of the day before. Security Brain would make *damn sure* to drive home the lesson that sleep was *bad*, sleep was *dangerous*. And she would keep me safely awake for as long as possible thereafter.

Imagine yourself to be a prehistoric human mother waking with the sun to discover that your babies have been dragged off and eaten by wolves. Now imagine you're in a hell where this scenario repeats itself endlessly. Each night in the wee hours, just when you can barely hold your head up, your babies reappear: sweet-smelling, dimple-kneed, immeasurably precious. You hug them to your breast, rocking them for a short while, then, overcome with tiredness, lay them on the mat; you tell yourself tonight is different, tonight there are no wolves, the pack has moved on; you lie down beside them and slide into oblivion. At dawn's first light, your eyes snap open to see ... two trails of blood flecked with gobbets of flesh, leading out the cave mouth. You scream and scream. Then the Devil himself shows up, in wolf form, all grins and slobbers and fetid breath: "This is what you *get*," he says, jabbing your chest with a crusty yellow claw. "This is what you *get* for falling asleep." He chortles and leaves you to your pathetic screaming.

Did I believe any of this was real? No.

Could I stop Security Brain from acting as if it were? Also no.

———

Morning. Walking back from ten a.m. meds run, I saw what appeared to be a meditation session going on in the circular yard by the cabins. Eight or ten clients were sitting on benches; another eight or ten were strewn about the flagstones, cross-legged or supine, hands resting on knees or chest, some in the sun, some in lacy patches of shade cast by the junipers. Standing at the center of the group was a woman with pigtails and an earnest demeanor, saying meditative things; behind her on the ground, a small boom box emitted new-age sounds while a vegetal clump in a burner emitted sage smoke. No thank you, I thought, and kept walking, but then I saw a massive white dog (*Great Pyrenees, maybe?*) wearing a red service jacket, sound asleep in a sunny spot. Nice-looking dog, I thought; maybe there will be dog interactions. I knew I wasn't supposed to be too close to anyone lest I spread my quarantine germs, so I found a spot on a bench in the back row, several yards from the goings on. I placed my purse between my feet and breathed.

After a minute or two, a woman with an air of author-ity joined me on the bench, leaning over to whisper through her floral-print mask, "Hi there. I'm Kendra, head of Client Operations."

"Jocelyn," I whispered back. "I got here yesterday."

"Welcome, Jocelyn. We're glad you're here."

"Thanks. Who is that in the middle?"

"That's Mindy. She's our alternative therapies counselor. She's great."

"Oh, I see."

"And that's her dog, Edith. Edith is a therapy dog."

"Oh, nice."

Mindy was now gesturing to one side of the circle and talking about "the East Gate." I recalled that on the daily schedule I'd seen something about a ceremony involving the four directions of Native American culture. I gathered that each direction, or gate, represented a part of oneself, or maybe a part of life. The East (Mindy was saying) represented beginnings, light, wisdom, I don't know what else; I was having trouble hearing, and besides, my attention was transfixed by Therapy Dog Edith and her impressive sleep skills. The humans seemed admirably relaxed, too, sitting on benches or lounging on the ground, all atten-tive to Mindy's smooth tones as she segued to the North Gate— which stood for "hardships, cleansing, endurance." Was there nobody here other than me who felt on the verge of a gibber-ing breakdown? The nurse at Unity had told me my new meds weren't here yet, they were on order from the pharmacy, which seemed like another setback, but, *they'll be here this evening. You just have to hold out till this evening.* Mindy transitioned to the South Gate: warmth, growth, plants in the earth. Could one pass through the gates? How close were the gates? A friend with a chronic illness had written on Facebook that you might be too sick to walk or even stand, yet health could be waiting for you in a world that lay no distance away, veiled by the thinnest of curtains. I wanted to believe this. I tried, as Mindy concluded with the West Gate—darkness, rain, end of life—and began waving the smoky sage around to the drone of the new-age music, I tried to *feel* the health that was there, just beyond the curtain or looking glass or through the low door in the wall, waiting for me to take one step, just one step in the right direction, and embrace it as an old friend.

It was no use. The only gate for me was the Sleep Gate, and that gate was barred.

————

After lunch. The early afternoon was taken up with a visit to my assigned therapist, Natalie, who wore a broomstick skirt and a pleasantly neutral expression. We sat in chairs placed six feet apart in a meeting room on the second floor of Harmony. I gave my account: vertigo, insomnia, anxiety, nerve pain, and so on and so forth. Natalie listened empathetically. She explained that I would have group therapy on Tuesdays, Thursdays, and Saturdays, and one-on-one therapy on Wednesdays and Fridays, but not this Friday, since I was officially in quarantine.

"That's all the one-on-ones?" I asked, disappointed. I had assumed they would be daily.

"You can request extra sessions, and I'll do them if there's time. We like to emphasize the group therapy, though."

"Ah. I see." *Listen, maybe group therapy will be good. Don't pre-judge.*

Of all the things Natalie said, I recall just two. First, she asked me if I knew about "relaxing your shoulders," prompting a small fit of internal hysteria as I thought about replying, *No I know nothing about relaxing my shoulders, but I do know all about deep breathing.* Second, she described the "adjunct therapies" on offer from outside specialists. One was a thing called EMDR, which stands for eye movement desensitization and reprocessing. "It's good for trauma," she said. "Many people find it helpful."

"OK ... I mean, I guess I am traumatized. Sure, why not."

"And we also offer horse therapy."

"Oh, wow! Can you actually ride the horses?"

"Well, no, but you lead them around. It's all about body language and trust. And leading."

"Oh."

"It's very popular. Only five clients per session. Would you like to do it?"

"Yes, please."

She handed me both forms to sign and said I should take them to the front desk right away and pay in advance with a credit card, because EMDR and horses tended to fill up. Sane Me blinked at the cost—in the hundreds for each program, non-refundable—but, *who knows, maybe it'll help. Take everything that's going.* I hurried over to Reception, once again congratulating myself on possession of my wallet. Kind Friendly affirmed the wisdom of my purchases as she swiped my card through the reader: "Oh, EMDR is amazing! It's really, really intense, but so great for trauma. And the horse therapy, you'll love it." As I walked back to my cabin, I reflected on the advantages of a captive customer base.

Still, everyone at the center was clearly wanting to help and trying their best. This was plain to me even as I sat in another group circle in another room in Harmony, Security Brain duking it out with Exhausted Brain while Natalie led a class that consisted mostly of her reading aloud to us, interminably, from a workbook about coping skills; even when I returned to the Unity meds room at four p.m. only to be told that I needed to fill out a separate insurance form for the pharmacy, which meant my meds wouldn't arrive for *another* 24 hours; even when, walking back from Unity, I came across Mindy leading a session on the picnic patio with Therapy Dog Edith, joined in, and discovered that Edith, while undeniably handsome, was a cold-hearted therapy dog, laser-focused on treats and impatient with fondlers.

Yes, I could see everybody meant well. It's just that I needed much, much more than well-meaning finger-snaps, or well-meaning counsel to relax my shoulders, or a well-meaning workbook about coping skills, or a well-meaning(ish) dog to snarf kibble from my palm. I needed medical treatment. And it seemed to me, as my first full day at the True Healing Center drew to a close, that the majority of my fellow inmates (*clients!*) were in better shape than I was; that this so-called healing program was serving, primarily, to keep them away from drugs and alcohol while they received help dealing with past psychological traumas, traumas that had led to self-loathing and self-sabotage. Of course they needed treatment, but mostly, I thought, they needed encouragement. *All have won, said the Dodo, and all must have prizes.*

I did realize I was better off than the fawn girl with her cutting scars; indeed, better off than all the fawn girls, three or four of whom, I came to learn, were housed in a building called Serenity and did not attend group sessions. At the nighttime meds lineup, one such girl would hunker on the weedy ground against the property's coyote fence, wrapped in a light blue blanket, her wistful face luminous in the moonlight. She and I discussed sleep aids: Seroquel, in her experienced opinion, was the best, while Trazadone she thought worthless. She told me Serenity was "where they put you if you can't ever be left alone. Somebody watches you 24-7." OK, I thought, I'm glad that's not me.

But the grownups, the cabin people: they all seemed in pretty decent shape. I envied their relaxed camaraderie. I envied their ability to sit at ease on their front porches reading books and waving to me as I walked by. I envied them their bright, reasonably well-rested eyes.

At five o'clock on Wednesday afternoon I was sitting on my bed, illicitly needlepointing an owl onto a change purse, when the cabin door rattled. Shoving canvas, yarn, and needle under my left hip, I snatched up my book of crosswords.

"Knock, knock!" came the cheery voice of CT Pat. "I've brought you a roommate!"

She entered, followed by the unhappiest-looking person I had ever seen.

CHAPTER 6

SONG OF THE MOCK TURTLE

~~~~~~~~~~~~~~~~

My intense irritation at having a roommate foisted on me melted within seconds into intense pity for the slump-shouldered woman in the entryway: lank blonde hair in a messy bun, wire-rimmed glasses circling red-rimmed eyes, nose sniffling as she watched CT Pat put down her bags and hang up her coat. Her features had a blurred, damp look, like paint rubbed with a sponge.

They had not gone far before they saw the Mock Turtle in the distance, sitting sad and lonely on a little ledge of rock.

"This is Kathy," said Pat.

"Hi Kathy! I'm Jocelyn."

"Hi." A scratchy whisper.

They must have already done Kathy's inventory, because Pat did not make her unpack or count off her possessions but went right to handing us the dinner menus. I marked my choices. Kathy stared at the sheet for a minute then said, "May I have a burger and fries?"

"Of course," said Pat. "Any vegetables?"

"No thanks."

"Anything to drink?"

"I guess a Coke."

I had gotten up in order to hand back my menu, so after Pat departed with a "See you ladies later!" Kathy and I were left standing side by side. She looked so lost, I forgot about the

104

no-touching rule and threw an arm around her shoulders, saying fiercely: "We're gonna get through this, OK? We're gonna get through this."

She didn't reply. I dropped my arm. She walked to her bed, pulled out her phone, and began to scroll, remaining on her feet with left hand tucked in the pocket of her fleece jacket. Her face was turned away, but I could see tears on her cheek. The sniffles continued.

> The Mock Turtle sighed deeply, and began in a voice sometimes choked with sobs, to sing:

> "Beautiful Soup, so rich and green,
> Waiting in a hot tureen!
> Who for such dainties would not stoop?
> Soup of the evening, beautiful Soup!"

Her sadness was a soupy, salty whirlpool whose dark suction I did not want to feel.

"Where'd you come from?" I asked, reseating myself on my bed.

"Michigan."

"Oh! That's a long way to come."

"Yeah." She kept scrolling. I picked up my crossword book. Eyes still on her phone, she said, "Sorry, I don't talk much."

"Don't worry, I completely get it."

"I also cry a lot." The way she said this, like someone mentioning that she also crochets a lot, took me aback; at the same time, the flat, why-should-you-care-how-I-feel tone was familiar. I had heard it coming from my own mouth.

Twenty minutes passed, and dinner arrived. Kathy sat down at the desk with her burger, fries, and Coke; I took my tuna wrap and carton of milk to my bed. Seeing some photos on her phone of what looked like children, I tried another conversational tack: "Are those your kids?"

A flicker of interest crossed her face. "Yes."

"How many?"

"Three. Two girls and a boy. Do you want to see?"

"Sure." I got up and went to look.

"That's Danielle, she's ten. This is Michael, he's seven. And Bethany—she's five."

"They're beautiful."

"They're the reason I'm here. I told myself I had to try again, for their sake."

"Have you been in other, um, centers like this one?"

"Yup. I've been hospitalized five times. Three suicide attempts. I have treatment-resistant depression. They think this place is my last chance, so I agreed to come."

"Oh, wow, I'm sorry." I returned to my dinner tray. I didn't want to hear more, but now she seemed inclined to chat and I couldn't very well get up and leave. On her cheeks the mock-turtle tears kept dripping, unwiped, as she continued in her scratchy monotone:

"I've been on like twenty different meds. The last time I was in the hospital they gave me ketamine. That's the stuff that makes you hallucinate for 24 hours. It didn't work. Nothing works. Now my docs want to try an MAOI, that's the old kind of antidepressant, but to do that I have to wean off everything else first, which takes like a month, and they have to monitor me the whole time, so I don't know. Maybe I'll do that."

"Yeah, maybe you should. Do you—do they know what the underlying cause is?"

"I was severely abused as a child."

"Oh, I see."

"Then I had a boyfriend who beat me up. Then after I got married I became a pediatric nurse, and I had this supervisor who kept assigning me babies born with addiction. I had six in a row. They all died. I told her I couldn't take any more babies, and I went out on sick leave, but when I came back and asked for a transfer, she said no, I had to take more babies. I couldn't deal with dead babies anymore."

She'll stop talking soon. She said she didn't talk much. She'll stop soon.

"So I quit my job. Now I basically just sit in my room all the time, and my husband brings me food. My kids are the only thing I keep living for. I want to get better for them." She glanced again at her phone. "But also, depression runs in my family. My nephew, he was eighteen, he jumped off a roof. Broke both his legs. Then they had him on suicide watch in the hospital, and he figured out he could lift up the bed and lay down and put his neck under the bed leg." Her lips curved in the slightest of smiles, as if to pay tribute to his resourcefulness. "He crushed his trachea. They found him like that."

I made no reply, for my mind was taken up with a brand-new idea: using a bed leg to crush one's trachea. In all my morbid musings, this possibility had not occurred to me. I envisioned the procedure: hoisting up the bed, wiggling underneath … I had to admit it was creative, but no doubt extremely painful, not to mention requiring immense upper-body strength and precision timing. No … no. Trachea crushing was really not an option. Not for me, anyway.

————

Around seven p.m., another newbie arrived. This one entered with a bang of the door and a gust of cold air, escorted by CT Lenora, who shouted, "You've got another roommate!" and left in a hurry. The new girl headed straight for the third bed, onto which she slung a large white plastic bag before facing us to say with a grin, "Hey, y'all! I'm Alicia."

"Hi Alicia, I'm Jocelyn, nice to meet you!" My brain churned in an effort to decide whether this development was good or bad. *Good,* said Sane Me. *Better not to be alone with Kathy.*

Kathy was lying stretched out on her stomach, propped on her elbows, feet at the headboard, several sets of colored pens strewn beside her. She was drawing hearts, flowers, and the word "GOD" in a spiral-bound notebook. She looked up, said "Hi," and resumed drawing.

Young and small-boned, Alicia had a freckled face and red-gold hair pulled back in a ponytail. She hopped onto her bed, crossing her legs. "So, where are y'all from?"

"Michigan," said Kathy.

"I'm from right here, Santa Fe," I said. "How about you?"

"Arizona," said Alicia. "Oh my god, what a trip. My bag got run over on the tarmac. All my clothes in it, shampoo, everything. Destroyed."

"What?! No way!"

"Yep. They just ran over it. All I have is my purse and this." She poked the plastic bag.

"But … that's horrible! You poor thing!"

"I know, right? I was like, *seriously?* This is all I need right now."

"God, I'm so sorry. Do you, uh, do you need to borrow some toiletries?" I was aghast. The thought of such a travel disaster was hitting me much harder than Kathy's dead babies.

"Oh thanks, no, I'm fine." She waved a hand. "They gave me some moisturizer and stuff. And they said they do Wal-Mart runs twice a week, so I can order more stuff then."

"OK, well, just tell me if you need anything. Did you get some dinner? I have protein bars and apples and … and some Triscuits." I'd received special permission from Dr. Funar, based on my too-low weight, to keep snacks in my room. I did not feel safe without my snacks and was loath to give any of them away, but clearly my food obsessions had to take a back seat to this dire situation. Had it been me with the squashed luggage … I couldn't even imagine.

"Yeah, I ate in the airport. Thanks, though." Stunningly nonchalant, Alicia pulled a slate-gray sweater from the plastic bag and put it on. She rummaged in her purse, found a pack of cigarettes, hopped off the bed and said, "Well, guess I'm gonna go to the smoke shack. Go be a dirty smoker! Ha-ha."

"Oh, ha-ha, sure! See you later."

She exited, leaving the plastic bag and her very small purse lying insouciantly on the quilt.

A little before eight she returned, bringing with her another burst of cold air and a smell of tobacco. She eyed me as she tugged off her sweater and said, "Are you doing needlepoint?"

"Yep," I said, holding up the canvas. "It's a change purse. With owls."

"Oh my god, that is so cute!" Flopping down prone on her bed, she took a paperback book with a black cover out of the plastic bag and began to read. For a while there was silence.

Then: "Hey, have you heard of this book?"

I looked at the cover but couldn't see the title. "What's it called?"

"The Subtle Art of Not Giving a Fuck."

"Ha-ha, that's great! Is it useful?"

"Yeah … I think so. I think it's helping me. This guy's a good writer."

"What are you in for, I mean, here for? If you don't mind my asking."

Alicia put down the book and sat up. "No, I don't mind. I slashed my wrists. See." She pushed up her sleeves to reveal white gauze bandages wrapped from wrist to elbow on both arms. *Vertical cuts. She was in earnest.*

"Oh," I said. "Oh, dear."

"Yep. I just took a knife and did it. I almost bled out. My boyfriend found me and called an ambulance. If he hadn't found me, I would've died."

"Oh, wow! Good thing he found you."

"I know, right? I'm really lucky."

"When was this?"

"Two weeks ago. First I was in the hospital. Then they put me in this place where I was on suicide watch and all the other people were, like, talking to the walls. It is *scary*. You're locked in and you can't have *anything*, no shoelaces, not even a pen, and they watch you all the time. The food *sucked*. I was there for four days."

"Jesus."

"But then my mom went online and found this place." She stroked one of the white bandages with a fingertip. "It's so pretty here. The sky is amazing."

"Yeah, Santa Fe is pretty. Do you, um, were you diagnosed with depression?"

"Yep, and meth addiction. I used to be into coke, sometimes heroin, and then my boyfriend was like, 'Do you want to try something that's a lot cheaper than coke and an even better high?' and I was like, "Hell, yeah!' That's how I got into meth. It was good at first." She stroked the bandage again. "But it kinda got out of control."

"How old are you? If you don't mind my asking."

"I'm twenty-six."

"Huh. My daughter is just three years younger than you."

"Oh, really? That's nice."

This whole time, Kathy continued to lie on her stomach, drawing hearts and flowers and GOD in her notebook, not saying a word.

————

On Thursday morning I attended my first group therapy session, which consisted mainly—and uselessly, from my perspective—of people presenting their "projects." Roommate Alicia, who seemed wondrously hip to everything despite having arrived only twelve hours ago, had clued me in as we ate breakfast: "Oh yeah, there are these projects we have to do, didn't they tell you? You're supposed to get the instruction sheet from the nurses' station." No, I said, no one told me. I rushed over to Unity to pick up the sheet and studied it as I sped along the asphalt path to Harmony, not wanting to be late. There were, I read, three projects, each requiring you to prepare a presentation on some aspect of your troubled past and/or plans for the future, using whatever "media" you wanted. As I entered the room and found a seat on a floor cushion next to Perky Daphne, I wondered whether laptops and projectors were provided for these media presentations. But "media," it would soon become clear, meant butcher paper and crayons.

The night before—with the help of my self-supplied Ambien (they'd located my missing pill bottle, thank goodness), an eye mask, and earplugs—I had managed to conk out for a full five hours, undisturbed by the bubbling wheeze of Kathy's CPAP machine; as usual, though, the sleep had been a fitful coma rather than a refreshing rest, and the dual morning claws of fear and exhaustion were clamped on my brain, rendering my memories of the group session blurry. I recall introducing myself and telling, briefly, about the vertigo and insomnia. And I recall two or three people presenting their so-called timeline project, an illustrated narrative of incidents in their life that had led them to this place of healing. Bill, a barrel-chested older man with a gruff demeanor, had a scroll of butcher paper ten feet long with events and dates meticulously noted in various colors. He asked for a volunteer to hold an end; no one responded for a few seconds, and I was just getting to my feet (*cooperative!*) when a dark-haired woman in a plaid flannel shirt stepped up. They stretched the scroll between them as Bill told his story:

In 1995 he began drinking. His son was born. He drank some more. His first wife left him. He drank some more. His second wife left him. He lost his job, joined AA, got sober, fell off the wagon, and lost another job. He moved to Colorado. His third wife left him. He scouted out a bridge, but the railing was too high to permit jumping. He got a DUI and wound up in jail, whereupon his son staged an intervention, "… and here I am." Finger snaps.

I also recall the flannel-shirted woman, whose name was Teresa, talking at some length about her rape. She had gone, she said, to a hospital for some type of emergency treatment, and while she lay semi-conscious in a curtained cubicle, in the middle of the night, a male nurse had assaulted her. "I was drugged," she said, pounding a fist on her thigh, her voice strident with emotion. "I could not stop him. I reported it to the hospital, but they would not believe me. They told me I had imagined it. I did *not* imagine it! He *raped* me. I was *raped.*" The men in the room looked uncomfortable; most of the women made moues of sympathy and murmured *we support you.* I think I simply looked at the floor. Teresa did not present a timeline, but she commented at length on other people's: telling them how far they'd come, how she felt their pain, how she loved them, then segueing back to her own story to revel in the progress she, too, had made. "When I first got here" (her finger jabbed toward the floor) "I could not even leave my room! Now look at me! I am healing! Praise Jesus, I am strong! I am not afraid!" On and on she went until finally the group leader said something to the effect of, "All right thank you Teresa, but we need to give everyone a chance," causing her to subside.

Poor Teresa, I thought. She lacks boundaries. Plus, she was raped. Me, I have too many boundaries, and I wasn't raped. *Exactly,* Sane Me snapped. *You have no excuse, none.*

Back at the quarantine cabin, Kathy, Alicia, and I ate lunch together, sitting on our beds with our trays before us. Kathy seemed in better spirits today. "What I want to know is," she said, taking a bite of apple and gesturing to the little heap of yarn and canvas next to me, "how'd you get them to let you keep that needle?"

"The CT never saw it," I said. "I smuggled it in. It's my illegal needlepoint, ha-ha! You guys better not rat me out." They chuckled and promised they wouldn't. "But what I don't get," I went on, "is why they confiscated my pencil sharpener. I mean, is anyone seriously going to take a pencil sharpener apart to get the razorblade so they can try and kill themselves? C'mon."

Kathy raised her brows as she took another bite of apple. "You'd be surprised," she said, chewing. Yeah, I thought, I probably would be.

After lunch Alicia and I set off for "Halloween Origami!" as announced in the daily schedule. We asked Kathy if she was coming. "No, I think I'll hang out here," she said, once again head-down with her notebook and pens. We walked over to Creativity, home of the crafts room, a small but light-filled space containing a long table flanked with chairs, counters laden with art supplies, and stacks of plastic drawers and bins stuffed with more art supplies. A dozen people were already there: Cool Kids Cameron and Jack, Perky Daphne and Silent Delia, Gruff Bill, Statuesque Janet, Emotional Teresa, and others whose names and faces I was starting to recognize. Leading the session was Marilynne, the activities director, a forthright woman with corn-rowed hair and an impressive ability to convey YouTube video instructions in real time. As we found seats she was standing at the table's head, passing out squares of blue origami paper; she proceeded to lead us through the construction of a bat—as in, nocturnal flying mammal—tapping her phone every few seconds to pause the video and demonstrate the next move. "OK, now you're gonna fold *this* corner to *here*. Like this, see?" She maintained a brisk pace, forcing us to focus. I was quite chuffed at how my bat turned out but, again, unsure as to the purpose of it all. *Twinkle, twinkle, little bat,* said Sane Me. *Keeping you busy, that's purpose enough.*

When Alicia and I returned to Number 1, we showed Kathy our origami creations. Alicia, laughing, joggled her bat to make its wings flap and said, "Seriously? I mean, Marilynne is great, everyone says she's the best staff person here" (I had figured out that "everyone" gathered and gossiped at the smoke shack, which accounted for Alicia's incredible savviness), "but, like, shit, I didn't come here to do second-grade craft projects. Look, Mom, I made a bat! Puhleeze." She rolled her eyes, but she placed her bat carefully on her bedside table. I did the same with mine. And Kathy opined that the bats were cute.

As dinnertime approached, we had a conversation about drugs. We began with our opinions on sleep aids (an extremely popular topic in Madland), which led to Alicia explaining why Xanax was her favorite before transitioning to the merits and demerits of heroin, fentanyl, and other opioids. "Fentanyl is baaad news," she said, dandling her cigarette pack on her knee, "and these days the heroin is usually cut with it, so you gotta be careful."

I poked my needle into Baby Owl and drew the yarn through. "The thing is," I said, "at this point I'd try anything, literally *anything*. But I wouldn't know how to get it! Like, where do you go to buy heroin? You can't just run to the store."

"Right?" said Kathy, looking up from her sketchbook. "I've thought about it, too, but what would I do? Drive downtown and ask someone on the street? Wave money out the window?"

"I guess you have to know a dealer or someone," I said.

"Yeah, I guess so."

"Maybe your friends refer you."

Alicia broke in. "Oh my god, you two are hilarious. 'How in the *world* would I ever buy drugs?' Too funny." She shook her head, grinning, as Kathy and I looked at her sheepishly. Then all three of us roommates burst out laughing, together.

———

Ten p.m., and my new medications still hadn't arrived. At the dispensary window, I swallowed my Ambien. I also received my estrogen patch (change twice weekly), unsure whether I was supposed to lift up my shirt to apply it under scrutiny, but, "You don't need to put that on here," said Nurse Tyrell, "you can take it back to your room." Tall, skinny Tyrell, though his zestful energy could sometimes turn flustered, was my favorite meds nurse. He liked to chat, and he always complimented my "great hats." In fact I had just one hat, a straw one decorated with plastic seashells, but I appreciated the sentiment. *Humanity. It's all about humanity.*

That night in the darkened cabin I lay in bed, eye-mask on, earplugs inserted, waiting for the Ambien to kick in. Ambien sneaks up on you like a tiger; though wide awake now, I knew in thirty minutes I'd be out cold. Alicia, I could tell, was also awake. Dr. Funar had prescribed her gabapentin, a non-addictive anti-seizure drug that is said to help with sleep, but it didn't seem to be working for her. She was tossing and turning, letting out a sigh now and then. Kathy was snoring loudly, having forgotten to wear her apnea appliance. At one point I got up, went to her bed, leaned over, and patted her shoulder: "Kathy. Kathy."

"Hmm ... mmpf ... wha?"

"Don't you need your CPAP machine?"

"Uhhh ... probably."

She rolled over and recommenced snoring. I tiptoed back to bed.

The thing about most sleep aids, I reflected, is that they don't make you any less sad or scared but merely drop a thick blanket of drowsiness on top of your scared sadness, transforming you from Grumpy or Bashful into Sleepy-Grumpy-Bashful, the Groggy Dwarf Who Is Still Awake. SSRIs and benzos, now: they are designed to treat two of severe insomnia's most common underlying causes, depression and anxiety, hence are often more effective. So why aren't SSRIs and benzos prescribed for insomnia more often? Well, SSRIs do get prescribed for sleep disorders, but because they tend to work over the long term and not so much in the short term, many doctors don't like using them for what might be just a short-term problem; also, because of SSRIs' often-unpleasant initial side effects, many patients don't stick with them long enough to help. As for benzos, they're hab-it-forming (some say addictive), so doctors prefer they be taken only for the mitigation of occasional, acute anxiety, not as a reg-ular thing.

I knew all this, yet what with Alicia's praises of Xanax and Dr. Funar's assurances, I had pinned a lot of hope on the clonaz-epam that I'd been prescribed along with the Zoloft. Surely, I thought, the new meds will fix me up. They will, right? *Yes,* said Sane Me with a firm, motherly nod, *the new meds will fix you up. You just have to hang on.*

Friday morning there was another crafts session led by Marilynne. This time, she handed out brown paper bags and proceeded to convey YouTube instructions for sticking onto our paper bag a face, a hat, a neckerchief, a shirt, and strips of yellow construc-tion paper (representing straw) in order to create—it took me a good 20 minutes to realize the end game—a scarecrow puppet. *Seasonal themes are very big here.*

The atmosphere around the table today was convivial, with chatter made possible by bag puppets' forgiving nature, totally unlike the intensity of origami bats. Cool Kids Cameron and Jack were seated across from me, sassily trash-talking each oth-er's artistic choices. Bill and his fellow gruff guys were taking it all in stride, exuding a gotta-get-with-the-program stoicism as they snipped and pasted. Alicia was down the other end, to Marilynne's right, looking young and tired. And Kathy, I was glad to see, was there too, in the chair to Marilynne's left; she had resumed her mock-turtle vibe—slumped shoulders, glazed eyes, surgical mask to cover her sniffling nose—but she went through the process as directed, rubbing a glue stick with slow care on each accoutrement before pressing it down on her brown paper bag.

People made idle remarks about what they'd eaten for break-fast, about their hobbies and hometowns, about the infuriatingly long wait for meds last night. Some laughed, shaking their heads ruefully at their creations: "Look at his mouth, it's deformed!" "Oh crap, my hands keep falling off." The scene brought to mind an old-time summer holiday camp, something from the 1960s, when entire families would go to the mountains to live in rustic cabins, play silly games, drink loads, and be otherwise entertained while fraternizing and/or fornicating with like-minded folks for a month or more, as in the movie *Dirty Dancing*. The difference here was that there was no dancing, no alcohol—and certainly no sex. (One of the many forms I'd signed at check-in had included the line, "I will refrain from masturbation.")

Still, the mood was jolly. Until, that is, someone asked Kathy a question, I didn't hear what, maybe it was about her intentions for the day, and due to one of those sudden silences that sometimes descends upon a group of talkers—whether by chance or, some say, the result of an angel passing through the room—Kathy's answer, delivered in the most dreadful, leaden tone of despair, was audible to everyone:

"I just want to know if I'll ever feel happy again."

The silence continued for a couple of breaths. Then Teresa, the rape survivor, spoke up: "You will. You *will*. I *know* you will." Kathy stared straight ahead. There were a few quiet "we support you's" from here and there around the table; then we all, including Kathy, turned our attention back to our scarecrow puppets.

———

My new meds arrived, finally, at eleven a.m. In anticipation I had made out an elaborate schedule for what were now six drugs and five supplements, and I showed it to the meds window nurse, asking if she approved. She did. I had the clonazepam down for six or seven p.m. each day, four hours before the Ambien to be safe, and the Zoloft for nine in the morning, but I went ahead and took half a Zoloft right then because Dr. Funar had said I could take it anytime.

When I got back to the cabin Kathy and Alicia were there, talking of this and that. Kathy, though positioned as usual on her stomach, propped on her elbows with her phone, sketchbook, and colored pens scattered around her, seemed much more animated than before; a little *too* animated, I thought, recognizing the signs of an adrenaline surge in her lightly flushed face, rapid speech, and nervous chuckles. Alicia's arm wraps had been replaced with smaller bandages; she unpeeled one of them to show the knife wound, saying, "I thought it might be getting infected, it's kinda red, see? So I went to the nurse, but they said nah, it's fine, it's healing well." I got up to take a closer look, fretting that "they" might be dismissing early signs of sepsis that would lead inexorably to gangrene, amputation, and a hideous death, but the thin red scar (hatched with tiny black stitches, like a zipper) did indeed look to be healing. *Kinda weird how you're so disturbed by some things and not others,* remarked Sane Me. *Suicide attempts, dead babies, rapes: whatever. Squashed luggage and a possible skin infection: the horror!*

At about one p.m. I went for a walk, circling the property as I calculated time (six laps, a quarter mile per lap, five minutes per lap, good, that'll be half an hour consumed), ending up at the center's forlorn, weedy labyrinth, which, if one wanted to stay with it, required an awkward crouch-and-scuttle under spiky juniper branches protruding over its northern edge. "Please maintain SILENCE as you enjoy this place of contemplation," said the sign; an unnecessary plea, since there was never anyone there but me and the only time I felt inclined to vocalize was when the junipers were scratching my face as I ducked underneath. The labyrinth took a good quarter hour to traverse, though, so it was worth a few scratches. After that I went to Summit, a.k.a. the cafeteria, and got a cup of mint tea. I did a few more circuits of the property, sipping gently so as not to burn my mouth, and then: Two o'clock! Time for a meds run.

On the benches behind Unity I joined Teresa and a new arrival, Andy, clearly of the gruff-guy type. As I sat down, Andy was griping about the program. "I came here for *therapy*," he said, "not to meditate and make puppets. I dunno. I might just leave. I dunno if this is the place for me." I asked him if he'd seen Dr. Funar, hadn't he liked her? "Oh, yeah, Dr. Funar is great," he said, "but that therapist they assigned me? I dunno." I shook my head in solidarity.

The previous client emerged, and Andy went in, leaving Teresa and me on the benches. Teresa said she understood Andy's feelings, but in her opinion he ought to stay, because "the program works if you work it. Look at me! When I got here I could not leave my room."

"For sure," I said, thinking that Andy was going to have a hard time adjusting. *Look at you, though; you made a bat and a scarecrow, didn't you? You're doing all right.* The Zoloft was having no discernable effect so far, but that was fine, I hadn't expected it to, it takes at least two weeks, it works if you work it. Teresa continued to talk about her successes while I watched the mountain air shimmering through the pine needles.

Then there was a crunch of gravel ... and Kathy came around the corner.

We waved hello to her as she approached. "Hey, Kathy, how's it going?" She sat down on the bench next to Teresa, jammed her hands into her fleece pockets, and closed her eyes. She was shaking from head to toe.

"You OK?"

"No," she gasped. "No. I'm not OK. I'm not OK."

If you've never had a full-on panic attack, you cannot imagine the intensity of the feeling that overtakes your brain and body: the sense that you can't breathe, can't speak, can't think, that you're free-falling into an abyss from which there will be no return. "Fight or flight response," the doctors say, but that really doesn't cover it. Having had panic attacks since the age of fifteen, I could imagine Kathy's feelings all too well. I stared at her, thinking of her agitation which had been evident an hour ago, thinking that I had foreseen this. She continued to sit, eyes tight shut, whole body quaking. I considered playing the savior, coaxing her to walk around the property with me for as long it took for the attack to subside; my own anxiety, however, was already rising up to meet hers, and all I wanted was to get away so I wouldn't have to witness her desperate state, so familiar, yet so strange when viewed from the outside. *Anyway, maybe this is something more serious, and she needs medical attention,* Sane Me cautioned. *You're not a doctor, honey bun.*

Teresa had placed a hand on Kathy's arm and was exhorting her to "breathe. Deeep, slooow breaths." She breathed and Kathy breathed with her, but it was obviously no use. "You're going to be OK," said Teresa, over and over, but Kathy was crying now, big mock-turtle tears leaking from her squeezed-shut eyes, and I could see there was no chance of her being OK for a bad long while. Nevertheless I joined in with the consoling, reaching out to pat her knee as she sat there, feet tucked tight under the bench, hands jammed into pockets, shaking and weeping. When at last Andy emerged, Teresa and I urged Kathy to go ahead, go ahead of us, go now. She rose with a hoarse "thanks," climbed the wooden stairs, and disappeared within.

"Oh my god," Teresa said. "Poor thing. Poor thing."

"Yes," I said. "Yes. Poor thing."

Teresa grabbed my hands and said, "Let's pray for her." I was busy trying not to think about what had just happened and I did not want to pray, especially not with hot, dry hands clutching mine; nevertheless, I bowed my head as she began: "Lord Jesus, we ask that you heal Kathy, that she may know your love, help her feel your love . . ." On and on Teresa prayed, with increasing fervor. I willed myself not to pull away. My straw hat was making my forehead itch, and the vertigo waves were swelling.

Suddenly she broke off, gripped my shoulders and squeezed. "I can *feel* your dizziness!" she said. "I *feel* it. Praise Jesus. I *feel* it!"

I froze, hating her. No you don't feel it, I thought; you don't feel it at all. And even if you did feel it, if Jesus himself felt it, if all the gods in heaven and earth joined me on my everlasting boat and shouted, "Feel the rhythm, feel the rhyme!"—how would that help me?

After getting to the meds window and swallowing my acyclovir, I did a few more laps around the property then headed back to Number 1, where the midafternoon light was slanting through the blinds and the air was cool and fresh. Strewn on Kathy's bed were her pens, sketchbook, and phone. I looked at the book, which lay open: more hearts, flowers, and GOD, all drawn freehand with skillful shading and 3-D effects. I sat down on my bed and picked up my coloring book and pencil box. Probably, I thought, Kathy would be back in an hour or two, dosed with an anxiolytic; either that or they'd put her in Serenity, the place where the fawn girls lived and were watched over 24-7. On my circular marches that day I had seen one of the fawns, a brunette, having a cigarette while perched on the concrete shelf that stuck out behind Serenity twenty yards up the prickly wooded slope by the walking path. Bathed in sunshine, crowned with wisps of smoke, she looked like a princess in a tower. The first time I passed I waved to her, but she didn't appear to see me, or at any rate, she didn't wave back. On subsequent laps I ignored her. What did the fawn girls do all day long? I wondered now, leaning back on the headboard as I colored a bird's wing and tried not to think about Kathy. Did they play board games? Attend therapy? Knit? No, knitting required needles, which are sharp. Origami, maybe. Macramé.

The door banged and in came Alicia. "Oh my god, did you hear? About Kathy?"

"Yeah, I was there." I put down the coloring book and sighed. "I was out back of Unity waiting for meds when she showed up. She had a major anxiety attack. Teresa and I tried to talk her down, but she was too freaked out."

"I know, and they took her away in an ambulance!"

"Wait, *what*? An *ambulance*? To the *hospital*?"

"Yes! On a stretcher. The whole deal. She's not coming back. If they have to call an ambulance, they don't let you come back."

Whoa, whoa, that's bad, that's very bad, but stay calm, it wasn't you they took away, it wasn't you on the stretcher being loaded into the ambulance. You know how to cope with these things and Kathy obviously doesn't. You're not her. You're not her. Everything's fine.

"Oh, no!" I said, arranging my face in the proper look of concern. "That's terrible."

"Yeah. Can you imagine? Poor thing!"

"Yes, poor thing."

We eyed the items scattered on her bed. "I guess they'll pack up her stuff and send it to her," I said, doubtfully. "Like her phone and stuff."

"I guess," said Alicia. "We should probably just leave it, huh?"

"Yeah, I guess we better just leave it."

But after Alicia had gone off to the smoke shack to gather more news, I took the phone and placed it, carefully, in the Mock Turtle's bedside drawer.

―――――

Around seven p.m. I went back to the meds window and asked for my clonazepam: 0.25 milligrams "as needed," as Dr. Funar had prescribed. The nurse chopped the pill in two with her tiny pill-guillotine, and I swallowed the pink semicircle along with another blue-striped acyclovir capsule. Then I returned to the cabin, where I sat and did a crossword while waiting for the drug to kick in. At last, at last, the good stuff! The silver bullet that would kill the beast!

Maybe not, whispered the tableau of abandoned items on Kathy's bed. *No, you're not like her,* Sane Me countered sternly, *you weren't abused as a child, you don't have treatment-resistant depression, you don't have a nephew who crushed his trachea with a bed leg. You're alert, cooperative, and well-groomed. And fundamentally sane. You're nothing like her.*

But the suspicion that I was like her, exactly like her, would not be shoved away. It nagged at me as I went on filling the squares of the crossword, monitoring myself second by second for the hoped-for effect of the pink pill, waiting to feel more calm—not totally calm, no, I wouldn't expect that, just a bit more calm—but instead feeling the small, sick, ever-present buzz in my stomach growing a little louder, a little stronger, a little bolder, until the tipping point came and a wave of fear whooshed upward into my brain and I heard my inner emcee welcoming a panic attack to the stage with the standard introduction:

Oh, no.

The wave flooded my body. I got up, grabbed my purse, pulled on my jacket, strapped on my facemask, and headed for the door. Counselor Mindy was holding a group session at seven-thirty with Edith the Therapy Dog; I hadn't planned to go, but they say petting an animal is good for panic attacks, and I'd never tried it, so, *Why not?* said Sane Me. My breathing automatically slowed and deepened as I hurried along the path to— Wellness, was it? I can't remember. My head swam, my limbs tingled, but I kept walking.

Perhaps oddly, I was less fazed by this boiling onslaught than by the three months of constant, simmering anxiety. A full-fledged panic attack is acute, not chronic; it lasts a couple hours at most, usually less. Besides, I'd lived through many such episodes, and I knew that the trick is—as G. Gordon Liddy once said as he held his palm over a candle flame until his flesh singed—"not minding." In this way, I really was unlike Kathy: a part of my brain was able to stand aside, observe the symptoms with dispassion, and above all, resist the temptation to try and make the attack stop. "You can't think yourself out of it," a wise doctor had said to me when at age 40 I hit perimenopause and the adrenaline fits started coming more often. "You either ride it out, or take something that'll shut it down." I'd chosen to ride it out, for although that doctor had willingly prescribed Ativan (another benzo) for such emergencies, I fretted there might be a bounce-back effect that would leave me in even worse shape, so I left the pill bottle in the linen closet and eventually threw it away. And now it appeared I'd been right not to take the Ativan, because the clonazepam had—obviously, no?—triggered this attack. As I entered the meeting room, although my body was overwhelmed with fear, most of my mind was seething with angry disappointment: *Dammit. The clonazepam didn't work. The silver bullet didn't kill the beast, it only riled it up. Dammit. Dammit. Dammit.*

A dozen people were already there, sitting in the folding chairs that ringed the space. Mindy was delivering a spiel about animal empathy and intuition as she walked the circle dropping a fistful of kibble into each hand, whereupon Edith (looking regal with her snow-white fur set off by her crimson jacket) would approach and bump the hand with her enormous wet nose. The kibble-holder would dispense the food bit by bit until it was all gone, causing Edith to move on to the next person, who would do the same. When she got to me, I tried to rub her soft furry ears between offerings: "Aw, Edith, what a good girl, what a beauty dog!" But Edith only twisted her massive head away with a snort of disgust and rammed my fist again with her nose. Chastened, I fed her the rest of the kibble bits in rapid succession.

Mad Me: I don't like Edith!

Sane Me: *Babe, I don't think Edith is in it for the likes.*

Mindy continued to hand out kibble while expounding on dogs' selfless love for all humanity. Edith continued to operate the human vending machines. My panic attack continued to whoosh, and I knew I couldn't sit still much longer—at least, I *could*, but only if I closed my eyes and remained absolutely motionless and mute, which would no doubt cause folks to stare, so I got up, approached Mindy and said in as polite a tone as I could force through my trembling lips: "I'm so sorry, but I'm going to have to go. I need to walk around for a bit."

"Oh, of *course*," Mindy said, with a look of profound sympathy that somehow managed, at the same time, to convey profound indifference. She must be used to this kind of thing, I thought as I exited. They're all used to this kind of thing. It's their job to be unperturbed by wackos.

Planning to make some circuits of the walking path, I headed across the parking lot and out the property's front gate. It was dark now, and if there was a fawn girl smoking cigarettes on the concrete shelf behind Serenity, I couldn't see her. Walking, breathing, walking, black sky above, black path at my feet, black prickly slope immediately to my right, black hulking hills far away to my left ... not a single light on the path ... being careful not to stumble in the dark ... then I arrived at the rear gate, the big black metal one, which was always left partway open during the day, and saw it had been slid across the gap. Shut. Locked. A new wave of panic swept me, but this time it was panic about something specific: When did they lock the gates at night? Didn't the rule book say eight o'clock? It was 7:55 now! What if they had locked the front gate just in the past few minutes?! I wheeled around and walked as fast I as could manage in the suffocating darkness, back the way I'd come, thinking that if the front gate was locked I could perhaps climb up the prickly slope, but no, there was a fence at the top, not a very sturdy fence, but still, was it likely I could even make it up that slope in the pitch dark? Of course I had my phone in my purse, good thing I took my purse everywhere, I could call someone to let me in, but it was after hours, no one was at Reception, no one would pick up, I didn't have anyone's cell phone number, then again surely they would hear me if I yelled, how embarrassing would that be, good lord don't let the front gate be shut, don't let it be shut, *please* don't let it be shut …

It was open.

I went through the gate, across the parking lot, and down the asphalt path to Unity. I went in the front door, up to the nurses' desk, and said to the air, "Hello. Hello. I'm having a problem."

A staffer approached. "Can I help you?"

"Yes, I took my prescribed clonazepam and it's not working for me. I feel worse. I feel really anxious." *Listen, do NOT give them the idea they should call an ambulance. They'll pack you off without your stuff and that'll be the end of you. Act normal. Concerned, but normal.*

"When did you take it?"

"About—I dunno, forty-five minutes ago?"

"Oh, that's not long enough for clonazepam to take full effect. You should wait a bit."

"No, I mean, it triggered my anxiety."

"What dose did you take?"

"Half of a point-five-milligram pill."

Another staffer joined the first one behind the desk. She said, "That's a very low dose."

"Right, but I feel bad. I don't like it. I—I thought I should let you know."

The two of them looked at each other, then back at me. "OK," said the first one. "We'll make a note of it for Dr. Funar."

"OK, well … fine. Thanks." I turned around and left.

Arriving back at Number 1, I found Alicia reading *The Subtle Art of Not Giving a Fuck.* I took off my jacket, put down my purse, fished a protein bar out of my tote bag, and settled down on my bed. I was starting to feel better—a good deal better, in fact. Maybe the locked gate scare had steered me off the unspecified-panic path. (*Or here's a wild idea, maybe the clonazepam is working.*) As I munched the protein bar and sipped a carton of milk I'd cadged from the cafeteria, I asked Alicia about her family. She was happy to talk about them: her mom, her brother, ordinary people living ordinary non-dysfunctional lives. She asked me what I was in for, so I told her about the vertigo and anxiety; she said, "Well that sucks!" I told her about my daughter and my books. We talked about Donald Trump. We talked about Kathy.

Before she headed off for her nightly smoke, she said, "I'm really glad I have you as my roommate. When I came here, I thought they might put me with some crazy person."

"Aw, thanks," I said. "Back atcha."

In the dawn, after another night of agitated semi-coma, I walked over to Unity and filled out the form to tell them I was leaving. By law they could not keep me, but twenty-four hours' notice was required if I wanted to reclaim my roller bag and, more important, my meds. I handed the form to a staffer; unfazed, she said she would tell Dr. Funar, with whom I'd have an exit interview that evening.

"Here, you need to sign this, too. It says you're leaving against medical advice." She pushed another form across the counter.

"Do I get my roller bag back now?"

"After dinner."

"And when do I get my meds back?"

"Who's picking you up in the morning?"

"My husband."

"So, when he gets here, load all your stuff in the car, be all ready to go, then come and tell us and we'll walk you out with the meds. We have to walk you out and put the meds straight in the car. We can't give them to you directly."

"Got it." I signed the medical release form without reading it and left.

OK so now you need to call Matt and tell him, and you need to pack, and you need to make it through twenty-four more hours in this horrible looking-glass house, but will it be any better at home? At least you'll get to sleep, or rather, NOT sleep in your own bed … "Hey, Jocelyn!" I turned to see Nurse Tyrell waving at me. He was heading cross-campus past the smoke shack, and without breaking his gangly stride he shouted, "Covid test came back! You're all clear!"

"No more quarantine?"

"Nope! You're good to go! You can go anywhere you want!" He flashed a thumbs-up and continued on his way, while Sane Me took a moment to appreciate the irony.

That last day, Saturday, was light on substance. In the late morning, Marilynne led some improvisation exercises in which I was asked to scream at someone, so I did, literally screaming *GAAAAAAAAH,* and everybody laughed because apparently that was not what was meant by "scream at." Cool Kids Cameron and Jack, taking advantage of a warm spell, sunbathed in shorts on the concrete terrace next to Unity; others worked on their projects in the crafts room; and I ate in the cafeteria for the first time, chatting with all the nice folks while feeling like a fraud because they didn't know I was leaving. (I had told only Alicia and one other inmate, a middle-aged woman who also had an odd neurological disorder, with whom I'd shared a few walks and conversations.) After lunch, I joined an outdoor yoga-aerobics session, again led by Marilynne. This was followed by an indoor Zumba video class that left me dizzy, aching, and demoralized by my inability to keep up with what once would have been an easy dance routine, not to mention annoyed by Teresa's shouting as I staggered breathless from the room: "Wow, Jocelyn, look at you doing Zumba! Look at the difference from when you first got here! You go, girl!"

Yes. This girl is going.

After dinner, Roberto came by to deliver my roller bag and stayed to chat. I sensed his disappointment in me. "The program works if you work it," he said, leaning on the portale post outside the door of Number 1. "It's helped a lot of people. I went through it myself, and I'm three years sober, so I know it works." Far behind him, dusk was starting to blur the foothills of the Sangre de Cristo. Unable to cope with his testimony, I said I had to pack.

At eight p.m. I went for my exit appointment with Dr. Funar. The movie *Beetlejuice* was being shown in Vision; seasonally appropriate music and merry laughter wafted through the night as I entered Unity and presented myself at the nurses' desk for the last time. *How many of those laughers are faking it?* I wondered. *Faking it like me and the Mock Turtle. Most, I bet.*

Dr. Funar welcomed me once again into her messy office, her Cheshire Cat smile in place, and expressed gentle dismay that I was going so soon. "I see you didn't like the clonazepam?" she said, consulting the notes in my file. "What was the problem?"

"It made me anxious. I had a bad reaction. And I don't see why I should take an addictive drug if it's not going to help, I mean, that seems counterproductive, right? Why would I take an addictive drug if it's just going to make everything worse—"

"No, no, of course not. We don't want you to take any medication you don't want to take."

Sane Me: *Hmm, I wonder whether we might—*

Mad Me: Shut up! We're leaving!

"Yeah, I definitely don't want any more clonazepam. But I will keep on with the Zoloft. I know it'll take a while to work."

"Yes, it can take a few weeks. No side effects from that? No nausea, headaches?"

"I don't think so."

"That's really good, that means you're tolerating it well. Remember, you're just on a baby dose right now. It's important to build up gradually to the effective dose."

> **Sane Me:** *You know, if we just think about this for a sec—*
>
> **Mad Me:** Shut up! Shut UP! I hate it here! Everyone is stupid and I feel horrible and I am going home! I do not like clonazepam, I do not want it, Sam I Am!
>
> **Sane Me:** *OK, OK! Stop shouting. You're going home, no one's stopping you.*

We talked for a few minutes about other sleep aids that might work for me. Dr. Funar suggested I keep taking the Ambien and said I might also try gabapentin, the stuff Alicia was on. "It's designed for seizures, but it's used for many different things. It's very flexible, very safe. And quite sedating."

"Oh, that's good to know. I'll ask Dr. Ortega about that, thanks."

"Good, well …"

> **Sane Me:** *Time's up. Ask her if she'll still treat you after you leave.*
>
> **Mad Me:** She's not going to do that, why would she? She'll be booked up, all the psychiatrists are booked up because of the pandemic, plus she only spends half the day at that other clinic, and anyway she's probably angry with me for leaving against medical advice, they're all angry with me—
>
> **Sane Me:** *OH MY GOD, JUST ASK HER!*

So I asked her, and she said yes.

I didn't know it then, but that ask was the single best move of my entire trip through Madland. If I hadn't made the request, and if I hadn't persisted, later, in jumping through the intake hoops required by Dr. Funar's clinic to take me on as an outpatient, I'm not sure I would ever have escaped from the dungeon I was about to enter: a world-sized, God-bereft, Hell-administered dungeon, where the lights were never extinguished, and the storm demons never slept.

CHAPTER 7

CUNNING OLD FURY

The panopticon, conceived by a certain eighteenth-century English philosopher with a keen interest in punishments and rewards, is a prison with cells arranged in a circle around a central station from which a single guard has a clear view of each cell. *Panopticon:* "all seeing." Although the guard can't watch all the prisoners at once, their inability to know when they *might* be being watched is—according to Jeremy Bentham, the philosopher—the key to assuring their good behavior. They will be motivated to act, Bentham says, *as if* they were being watched. The panopticon concept was welcomed, initially, as useful not just in prisons but also in factories, hospitals, poorhouses, asylums, or anywhere humans seek to control other humans; no actual panopticon was ever built, however, and its Orwellian tinge caused it to fade from favor. Today, of course, we have Alexa.

I returned home from Looking-Glass House early on Sunday, October eighteenth. After helping Matt transport my luggage, weighted blanket, and giant baggie of meds-plus-pencil-sharpener-and-scissors from the back of the Jeep, I went straight to the bedroom, crawled under the duvet, and passed the rest of the forenoon in a torturous fugue state, Exhausted Brain and Security Brain waging a war in which I lurched at spasmodic five-minute intervals between nightmares that at least weren't consciousness and consciousness worse than any nightmare.

At lunchtime, Matt showed up bedside: "How are you feeling, Woolly Bear? You want something to eat?"

I opened my mouth, but no words would come. I wanted him to go away. I wanted him to climb into bed with me and hold me tight. I wanted him to bash me on the head or stab me through the heart. Anything, anything to make the reeling writhing sleep-wake agony stop.

I took a deep breath and tried again. "I ... I ... can't. I can't." A pathetic, scratchy whisper, just like the Mock Turtle's.

"How about some toast? A little piece of toast? Doesn't that sound good?"

"No ... uh ... oh ... OK."

"And a banana? Half a banana?"

"No ... OK ... yes. Banana please."

I forced down the food. Feeling as per usual slightly better as the day wore on, I took a shower and went for a couple of walks. The vertigo had worsened—more up in my head now than down in the ground—and the anxiety kept up its frantic toddler whine, but I was able to sit in the rocking chair and do an easy crossword, watch television, read a little. I couldn't do ballet barre exercises anymore, but I could sit on the floor and stretch. "We just need to wait it out," said Matt as I swallowed my bedtime pills, relieved not to be lining up in the cold for the Unity meds window. "Wait for the drugs to work." He was happy about Dr. Funar and the Zoloft; I could tell he had decided it was his job to keep me on this prescribed medical path for as long as it took, and, *He's right,* said Sane Me. *You have your Ambien, your Zoloft, your estrogen patches. Nothing to do but wait. Things will turn around. Soon, soon, the prosecutor will say it was all a big mistake, that there's insufficient evidence to indict, and you'll walk free.* But next morning I woke before dawn to the snickering wolf-jailer jabbing me with his crusty yellow claw, the sick thrumming fear unendurable (yet I endured it), and in hindsight I see that the indictment was already in. I had been remanded without bail.

The panopticon-prison in which I spent the next seventeen days was the reverse of Jeremy Bentham's. It wasn't the prison guard but I, the accused, who stood alone in the well, chained, under harsh lights with demon watchers staring down at me: tier on tier of them rising upward as in a Greek amphitheater or Mad Max's Thunderdome. Matt was there, too: sometimes he was the warden, a kindly one for the most part but staunchly on the side of the Law and devoted to his carceral duties; other times he was a fellow prisoner, chained beside me, cringing in the interrogatory glare. Dr. Funar was my lead defense attorney, but an attorney who worked remotely and was reachable only by phone through a harried assistant. To her I was able to make a couple of calls a week, no more, to get her counsel, which she gave in the form of additional prescriptions—a higher dose of Zoloft, an additional sleep aid—plus encouragement to wait, wait until the drugs took effect. I asked her, once, if I should go to the hospital. "No," she said, "they'll just give you the same medications and release you after a day or two. You should stay home, where you have more control."

More control? How can I have *more* control when I don't have *any* control? Tell me, Doctor, what must I do to regain a shred of control? On the other hand … Don't you tell me what to do, *I'm* in control. Dear Doctor, God, Universe, Somebody: Give me control. Please, please, give me back my control, which I have mislaid and fear I will never see again.

———

Then there was my defense team: the people who were making efforts, each in their own way and according to their own capacities, to help me through the trial. They clustered in three groups: friends, family, and healthcare professionals. Many had been leaning in for some time, having either heard from me directly or read my occasional "Hey check out this crazy medical mystery!" Facebook posts. Each one listened; each one cared; each one offered analysis, assistance, or advice. None, alas, could offer a solution.

There was my friend Margaret in Austin, Texas, who said she'd come to Santa Fe and take me on holiday to a restful retreat in the mountains (different mountains, that is). "You need a break," she said. "I'll make all the arrangements. Just say the word."

There was my former boss James in Boston, who due to his daughter's long bout with leukemia was an insider at all the top New England hospitals. "Get on a plane," he said. "Stay with us. I know loads of specialists, I'll get you in."

There were the Fellow Sicklings, as I thought of them: friends and acquaintances also suffering from weird chronic illnesses—autoimmune disease, Lyme disease, hormonal problems, traumatic brain injuries, ear issues, fibromyalgia, chemical sensitivity—who shared their experiences and tips. "Plant-based diet," said one. "B vitamins," said another. "TENS." "Low sugar." "Meditation." "SSRIs." "Marijuana."

There was Dr. Greene, the Caterpillar ENT, with whom I spoke again after developing a searing sore throat and, worse, a hypersensitivity to sound that had me wincing in pain every time a dish rattled or a car horn honked. I asked him over the phone if he'd give me an antibiotic for possible strep. "Ninety percent of sore throats are caused by viruses," he said. "It'll probably last a week or so. Take Tylenol: 500 milligrams three times a day is absolutely fine."

"What about the noise sensitivity?" I asked, holding the phone six inches from my ear.

"That's probably because of the virus. It'll go away."

"And the vertigo? I thought it was getting better but now it seems worse. More up in my head, less down in the ground. And I think that's making the insomnia worse."

"Hmm. I really can't link the vertigo to the insomnia. Well, unless lack of sleep is keeping your brain from adapting to the vertigo, thereby making it worse."

"Yes, right, so what do you think I should do? Is there a sleep aid you recommend?"

"No. Take Tylenol for the throat pain."

Oy … he STILL thinks you're a drug-seeker.

I called Dr. Ortega's office and badgered Nurse Practitioner Just-a-Nervous-Girl into prescribing me penicillin over the phone. "Have you had strep throat before?" she asked. Oh yes, I said. "And this feels the same?" Oh yes, I said. She sent the prescription in. I took one pill that evening and decided the time was right to immerse myself in a sea of internet opinions re: Why Antibiotics Are Terrible. Fully convinced, I added the penicillin to the raft of rejected pill bottles on the third shelf of the linen closet and shut the door.

There was Therapist Denise, with whom I continued weekly phone sessions in which I struggled to describe how awful I felt. "I want you to keep a dream journal," she said. "Write down your dreams each day. We'll talk about them." I told her that would be difficult, for the Ambien coma was dreamless and I couldn't remember much of the sleep-wake agony nightmares. "That's OK," Denise said; "whatever you can remember." I duly recorded three dreams, bad dreams all, in a fresh new forest-green Moleskine notebook that I unearthed from the office supplies shelf at the back of the basement.

There was Nurse Stephanie, who phoned me from somewhere in Maryland having been informed by the insurance company about my stay in a rehab facility. It was her job, apparently, to follow up with the head cases. "I'm here to help you however you need," she said in her young, light Southern accent. "You can call me anytime." Buoyed by the thought of my very own nurse-concierge, I asked her to help me with my latest mission: getting into Dr. Funar's outpatient clinic. "Sorry," she said, "I can't help with that." I asked her to explain some insurance puzzles. "Sorry, I can't help with insurance." I asked her if I should go to the hospital. "That's your decision; I can't give you medical advice." *Well, alrighty then.* Moreover, "call me anytime" turned out to mean: Call Monday through Thursday, nine to four Eastern, and leave a message. Stephanie was very sympathetic, though, and checked in with me faithfully twice a week. I dubbed her Stephanie the Nice-but-Useless Nurse.

There were my two big brothers, one in South Carolina, the other in Oxford, England. I had emailed them a week before when I was preparing to check into the True Healing Center, but I don't think I managed to convey the situation's gravity. "The surest sign of mental health," wrote back South Carolina Brother, "is knowing when you need help." "You're in Santa Fe," wrote Oxford Brother; "there's got to be someone around who can wave sage over you. What about Rolfing?" Once back home, I reported in again with a lengthy account of Why that healing place was a bad place. My South Carolina sister-in-law took over the family communications thereafter; she had me, she said, on their prayer list at church. When an alcohol reek began to rise from the basement and I realized Matt was drinking multiple glasses of wine at night so *he* could get some sleep, and that we *both* really needed a caretaker, I considered sending an S.O.S. to South Carolina, but didn't. Why didn't I? For one thing, I needed every ounce of willpower just to get through the aching, itching, bouncing, clanging, miserable terrified bug-eyed slow-motion marathon that each 21-hour day had become. For another thing, I didn't see the point. What could anyone do that Matt and I weren't already doing?

There was my friend Susan in Toronto, who phoned me regularly to check in and share ordinary news of what was going on in her life, until I asked her not to (listening became almost as hard as talking), after which she switched to chat messages bearing a note, a funny meme, an old photo of us together. "I'm still out here, lurking creepily!" she wrote. "I love you."

As for friends and neighbors in town: there were some who surely would have rallied round had I asked them—but I wouldn't have known what to ask. Also: Covid.

Last and most of all, there was our daughter Emily, now 23 years old, off at grad school in Texas. In the closing week of October I wrote her a letter in my Moleskine dream journal—a letter I never sent, though I marked it with an orange sticky note so she would find it in case, as seemed increasingly likely, I were to be "put away" somewhere—asking her to forgive me for leaving her and to remember me as the good mom I used to be. I told her to rely on Margaret, my Austin friend, who had promised to look after her. I told her I loved her very, very much. I hated to think of her worrying, so I hid my deterioration from her as best I could, but she knew, of course she did, and she offered to revive her early-pandemic practice of sending me a daily wakeup text: "Good morning, Mummy!" with an emoji, different every day—a heart, a flower, a cow face, a lion face. Each of those text messages was (how else can I put it but tritely?) a tiny ray of sunshine through a chink in my dungeon wall.

————

My entire defense team meant well; they tried their best. Yet I remained in the prisoner's dock looking at them looking at me, a wall of glass between us, the floor under my feet bumping down, down, like a janky elevator, taking me farther from aid and nearer to the executioner's block. What would I say to them now, other than "Thanks for trying"? What would I say to anyone who wants to defend a friend, patient, or loved one against the brutal encroachments of insanity?

When faced with a mentally ill person, few of us can resist offering advice. We tell the ill one to get outside, stick to a routine, engage in self-care, take supplements, see a therapist, go on vacation, come for a visit, or try Rolfing. We suggest they exercise, journal, breathe, meditate, knit, eat plants, or smoke weed. When we see our advice isn't landing, most of us know enough to back off: we revert to offering a sympathetic ear, a shoulder to cry on, support as requested. "Talk to me," we say. "Call me anytime. Let me know how I can help." And we're right to say those things. Listening, after all, is what a good friend does. But the critical point we tend to miss is that a person with major depressive disorder isn't "feeling down." A person with an anxiety disorder isn't "experiencing some stress." A person with obsessive-compulsive disorder isn't "so anal, ha-ha." A person with bipolar disorder isn't "moody."

A mentally ill person is *sick*.

Certainly as sick as someone with pneumonia, possibly as sick as someone with cancer. We don't expect a friend with pneumonia or cancer to chat to us; we don't expect them to feel better because we invited them out for a drink and encouraged them to share. We take their illness seriously, knowing that we as laypeople can't fix it, and we don't demand they perform wellness in order to ease our fears. A friend with a mental illness, though: while it's easy to understand, intellectually, that they're sick, it can be hard to grasp that they're *really and truly* sick, sick to a degree that all the sharing in the world won't mitigate. And of course the last thing we want is to be blamed, should worse come to worst, for not having done everything we could. So ... "Talk to me," we say. "Call me anytime. Let me know how I can help. Have you tried cannabidiol?"

What the mentally ill person hears: "Take responsibility, amid your illness, for creating the circumstances whereby I can help you." And now, for that mentally ill person, another task looms: another task in the overwhelming, minute-by-minute, breath-by-breath effort to bear the torment, which is fast becoming the only item on their agenda.

I expect I sound churlish. What else can people do, after all, other than reach out and listen? Do I not appreciate those who worried, who called or took my calls, who emailed or messaged as I was spiraling down the well? Am I not grateful to Margaret, James, and Susan, to the Fellow Sicklings, to Therapist Denise, to the brothers South Carolina and Oxford, to the nurses Nice-but-Useless and Just-a-Nervous-Girl? To Emily, who sent me good morning emojis of hearts and flowers, cow and lion faces? To Matt, who supplied endless mugs of tea and said, "If you're scared in the middle of the night, just come downstairs and wake me up, I don't mind"?

I am grateful. I am deeply, deeply grateful to every one of them. But not for the advice. Not for the offers of help. Not even, really, for the sympathetic ears. You know what I'm grateful for? *They were there.* They sat in the panopticon seats, scattered among the leering, heckling demons, and with calm, interested eyes watched my trial unfold. Their attempts at back-bench coaching were, quite frankly, ineffective; even their cries of encouragement or commiseration failed to make me feel better, because in the end, the only person who could make me feel better was me, along with serious medicine and (maybe) divine intervention. But their mere presence—*that* made a difference. The simple fact that they emailed, messaged, called, answered, invited, or shared their news, that they said, "How are you?" "I'm sorry," "Praying for you," "I love you," "Hey, remember when?" "Wow, that sounds bad!" or really *anything at all*—made a difference.

As it turns out, those friends and family, nurses and therapists, weren't my defense team. They were my witnesses. And witnesses, it turns out, by some mysterious mechanism make torment just a tad more bearable.

————

Saturday, the last day of October. Halloween.

At 3:47 a.m., the Ambien gives up the fight. I open my eyes to the unholy dark, reach for my phone, check the time (God have mercy) roll onto my back, and enter the sleep-wake fugue state. The ill winds gather strength, the bad waters creep up the levee as I lurch in and out of evil dreams, longing for oblivion, nothing more. After what seems an age, I check the time again: 4:05 (Shit god shit). The house is dead quiet except for the sporadic tick-tick-hiss of the steam radiators. Matt is asleep downstairs on the Magicouch. The air is frigid.

Last night about this time, I challenged the storm to do its worst: *Just lie here and breathe,* Sane Me instructed. *Let it rage. It might blow itself out if you let it rage. You can do it, I know you can! You're strong enough.* So I there I lay, letting wave after wave of hurricane-force anxiety wash over me, curled in a fetal position on my right side, head propped on three pillows, eyes shut tight. Sweat ran from every pore and wet my pajamas, then the sheets, as I used pure will to stay immobile with Elephant hugged to my breast, thinking nothing but *Breathe in ... breathe out ... breathe in ... breathe out ...* for what, 30, 60 minutes? The storm did not abate.

With that failed experiment of yesterday in mind, I sit up, snap on the light, and rummage beneath the duvet for my grain-filled microwaveable heating pad. I bought this beanbag-like item for Emily on Etsy, many years ago; since she moved away it has had a new life with me, warming my feet through the cold Santa Fe winters. It's the size of a baby doll's pillow, its brown cotton case stamped with white paw-prints. You're supposed to microwave it for one minute, no more; I always do a lot more. By morning the only heat it retains is body heat, but its texture is compelling nevertheless, and it still gives off a faint cooked-rice odor that I've come to perceive as pleasant. Now I cross my legs under the covers, put the beanbag in my lap and start to scrunch it with both hands, violently, over and over, as I rock back and forth, whimpering. Scrunch, scrunch, scrunch. Whimper, whimper, whimper.

Twenty-three minutes pass thus.

At 4:29 I struggle out of bed, walk sweat-drenched and shivering to the kitchen, obtain a small piece of bread and a banana, go back to bed, force down the bread and half the banana, then lean back on the pillows with the light on, trembling and scrunching, breathing in breathing out, eyes sometimes open sometimes closed, for another half hour. "This is what you *get* for sleeping," snarls the wolf-jailer. He has a whip now, and he doesn't hesitate to use it: "This! Is!" *Swish, Crack* "What! You!" *Swish, Crack* "GET!"

Please. No. Please, make it stop. God, make it stop. Somebody, make it stop.

At five a.m., I hear Matt coming up from the basement. I rise again and stagger to the kitchen. "Good morning, Bear!" he says, and holds out his arms. He's in his boxers and a ratty t-shirt, looking dead tired and smelling of wine and mildew. I resolved, last night, to take him up on his offer to comfort me when scared—*Maybe if you just shout it out, that's it, shout, shout, let it all out*—so I say, "Good morning," then fall on his neck and start literally yelling: "OH GOD, OHHH GOD, OH MY GOOODDD ..." This continues for perhaps 30 seconds. Sane Me, observing the scene from a vantage point somewhere above and behind my right shoulder, can tell that this shout-it-out business isn't helping and, moreover, that my husband is seriously unnerved; he's hugging me tight, patting my back, whispering, "Shush, it's all right, shush," but, *You're freaking him out,* says Sane Me. *Cease and desist.* I step back, releasing him, and he guides me back to bed, tucks me in, brings me a mug of mint tea.

"Try to sleep some more," he says.

"I can't. I can't." My body reeks of the flop sweat. I grab the tepid beanbag, place it on my chest: scrunch, scrunch, scrunch. The bedroom is icy: since the steam radiator busted a seal, years ago, we've used a roll-around electric kind, which is fine for brisk fall temperatures but relatively useless in a deep cold snap such as this, not to mention that the room's ancient crank-handle windows don't seal properly. Heavy snow is forecast for tomorrow, the first day of November. It's going to be a long, cold winter. (What about the woolly bears—the weather-predicting caterpillars? Their red bands must be extra thick these days)

"Here's your Kindle. Why don't you watch a movie?"

"I can't. No. No. I can't."

"What do you want to eat? You'll feel better after you eat something."

"Nothing. No. I don't know."

"I'm going to bring you some toast and orange juice. You want some oatmeal? Banana?"

"No. I had a banana. Some banana. I don't know. Toast. Yes. Thank you."

He brings me the toast and OJ. I thank him again then set about chewing and swallowing, chewing and swallowing. I know I need to eat, that I'll get even sicker (*ha, how is that possible?*) if I don't eat. When they weighed me at the Healing Center, I was 117 pounds. Dr. Funar said, as she placed the stethoscope to my chest, "Wow, you're so thin I can see your heart beating!" These days I probably weigh even less.

Around 5:30 I take a shower and dress. Deciding what to put on feels like lifting a barbell, but it's necessary to wear clothes in order to go out for a walk, which is what I'll be doing for most of the daylight hours, taking random routes around the neighborhood as my legs lead me, here and there, up and down, round and round, maybe six or seven miles in all. Like Forrest Gump. A week ago I had the weirdest sensation, brought on, I couldn't be sure, either by the increased Zoloft (now at 25 milligrams) or by the long-term Ambien: I felt as if I were walking through molasses, as if I'd entered some sort of Star Trek slo-mo dimension. The feeling wasn't exactly unpleasant; in a way it felt restful to be oozing along while everyone else was scurrying, and lord knows any form of rest is welcome, even if I have to get it while in motion, as sharks do. This morning, however, the molasses sensation has gone and I'm back to a moderate pace, restrained only by the constant, intense ache in every joint and muscle. *Your body is breaking down,* Sane Me observes mildly as I lock the kitchen door, make my way down the gravel driveway under the halogen glow of the streetlight, and turn left on Granada. *Soon you won't have the strength to walk at all, and then what will you do?*

I turn right on Booth Street in order to visit one of my trees.

Trees are a major focus these days. Hanging, I have decided, is the only feasible way to go, and what's needed for hanging (I reason) is a tree with a branch low enough to throw a rope around while I stand on a chair or fence or wall, but high enough (obviously) so my feet don't touch the ground after I drop. It's surprising how many trees are *not* suited to the purpose—almost as if God has designed trees, most of them anyway, to be suicide-proof. Kind of frustrating, to be honest. Nevertheless, there are four or five trees in the neighborhood that might do; this aspen-like one on Booth Street is especially promising, though it lacks a well-placed wall so will require me to bring a chair, which might be difficult, then again it's only a block from home, it won't be hard to carry over a small chair, or maybe the stepladder, plus the property on which the tree sits is an apartment complex, not a single-family home, which is good because I don't want to inconvenience a homeowner, but of course people *will* be inconvenienced, imagine looking out your window with your morning coffee and seeing a dead body hanging in a tree and you have no idea who it is and you have to call the police and it's a whole big thing, how rude is that? And how will they know whom to contact? I will have to write a note with contact info, put it in my coat pocket, I'll do that when I get back ... I wonder if anyone's looking at me right now, as I stand here on the sidewalk looking up at this perfectly nice innocent tree, this must be like the thirtieth time I've done this, stand and stare at a tree, surely one of the neighbors has seen me and knows what I'm thinking, how embarrassing! I should just do the deed at home, but no, no, can you imagine, Matt will be devastated if

I do it at home, poor guy, and anyway I've looked everywhere at home and there's no place that's any good except for the iron fence above the outside stairwell down to the basement, there's a nice drop there, but that rose bush is in the way, stupid thorny rose bush, never liked it. No, it has to be a tree. Still, when I get home maybe I'll have another look round the house and yard. For now, I'll keep walking. Keep going, go, go, *here it takes all the running you can do to keep in one place, said the Red Queen.* Turn left on Don Gaspar. There's another tree in this block, maybe two, that're worth assessment. This one, for instance, this one here has a good stone wall right next to it, let's climb up on the wall, must be careful in the semi-darkness, though ... up we go ... easy, now, hold onto the bark ... let's take a closer look at this big branch, see if it'll work. Hmm. Maybe.

I climb down and continue on the trek. Franklin, one of my dog friends, barks at me as I go past his gate, bringing startled tears to my eyes. Even the dogs hate me now. The sky is getting lighter. It's very cold. If I walked into an arroyo and took off most of my clothes and lay down, how long would it take me to freeze to death? They say freezing to death is quite pleasant; they say you get sleepy and warm and just drift away. Sounds OK. But the temp probably needs to be, like, subzero for hypothermia to set in fast, and what is it now, 20 degrees, 25, warming up to 45 once the sun rises at 6:30? That's not enough time. Maybe I could do it earlier, like at four a.m. *Right, like you'll have the willpower to get up, leave the house, and find an arroyo at four in the morning.* True, true, and suppose I did manage to do it and it worked and they found me half-naked, dead in an arroyo! That'd be even more embarrassing for everyone than the other scenario. No, no, it has to be hanging. Any other method is completely impractical.

Ten a.m. now, and I'm on my second walk—or is it the third? I am keeping a lookout not only for trees but also for other likely structures. Downtown there's a footbridge over the

Santa Fe River (dry at the moment, and it's hardly a river at the best of times, just a small stream) which has steel bar railings and, again, a nice drop. No need for a chair when there's a nice drop. I crouch down, patting the railings with my gloved hands, imagining how I will loop my scarf (yes, even though Matt confiscated most of my scarves at the bidding of Hotline Lady, I still have one, a lavender cotton open-weave, I'm wearing it now) around my neck, then tie it to the steel bar, then climb over—or would I have to climb over first, *then* loop and tie the scarf? It all seems extremely awkward and challenging. I am also vaguely aware that I do not know how to tie a proper noose, not really, and that the scarf is not long enough, and the fabric is not strong enough, and moreover *that I do not want to die.* But I go on planning and walking, walking and planning, examining the trees and footbridges and playground monkey-bars and basketball hoops and even the big metal outdoor sculptures that belong to a gallery at the bottom of Canyon Road, but mostly the trees, my stalwart friends, the trees—because as long as I am planning my suicide, as long as I am looking at trees, I am doing something to solve the problem. I have a focus, a purpose, a goal. I am seeking a way to Make. It. Stop.

Months later, Susan and I will laugh about it: how I would cruise the neighborhood for hours, soberly assessing the trees for hanging potential. "I bet you had them plotted on a two-by-two matrix," she says. "Oh, you bet," I say, "I had a whole spreadsheet!" Gallows humor, literally. But at the time, it did not feel the least bit humorous, or even all that crazy. Rather, it felt like managing a serious, vital project, like launching the Space Shuttle or negotiating with the Ayatollah for the release of hostages. A matter of life and death. And Sane Me (unbeknownst to Mad Me) was the project manager, the driving force behind this deadly serious planning.

"But," you object, "that can't be right. If someone has a suicide plan, that means they're closer to doing it, which is a very bad sign. Much worse than just thinking about it."

Yes, I'm sure that having a suicide plan is indeed a very bad sign. I'm not convinced, though, that *planning* suicide is at all the same as *having a plan.* The medical pros asked me many times whether I had a suicide plan; when I answered yes, what I meant was not that I had *a plan,* noun, but that I was constantly *planning,* verb. A plan is an executable file on your computer, sitting inert until you decide to open it: <Are you sure you want to run this program? Click yes only if you trust the sender> But plan*ning*—that's not a file you open, it's a process in which you engage, a process that may continue indefinitely.

When I'd called the crisis hotline a few weeks before, Hotline Lady suggested I think of some future event I could plan for and look forward to, such as my daughter's birthday or a family trip. Although this advice was no doubt sound, I was in such pain that contemplating anything beside the pain, how to endure it and how to stop it, really wasn't possible. If you're trapped in a burning building, you can't be planning a birthday party; what you can be planning, and should be planning, is how to douse the fire or exit the house. "Douse fire or exit house" was the very sensible assignment Sane Me had put on my plate, and since the heat was growing intolerable while all attempts to stifle the flames had failed and all ordinary routes of egress had been blocked, my new assignment was to locate the button that would blow the escape hatch. A twisted assignment, for sure, and perhaps a dangerous one. (Don't try this at home!) But as long as I was seeking the button not pushing it, compiling the file not clicking it, planning my death rather than carrying out the plan—I was staying alive.

————

Early afternoon, same day: I'm between walks, inside, looking out the window at the devil waving his arms and groaning.

This is not a hallucination. The residents of the house facing ours, half a block away where our little street meets the big one, are holiday decor enthusiasts, and this year for Halloween they have stepped it up a notch by placing in their front yard an eight-foot animatronic devil with a red robe, red ram's horns, fierce glowing red eyes, and a white-fanged, red-lipped mouth that opens and closes in a rictus grin while the vocals sync with waving arms: *BWAHAHAAH ... MWAAHAAHAAH*. This festive satanic figure is visible, day and night, straight out our living room window; for nighttime viewing, the homeowners have provided eerie lighting effects. Although their yard is walled, our property's slight elevation provides a nearly unimpeded sightline, and the devilish groans and growls are audible within a two-block radius: *BWAHAHAAH ... MWAAHAAHAAH*.

While Mad Me finds the display deeply unhelpful, Sane Me is wryly amused. *You have got to be kidding me!* she says, every time I walk past the hideous red robed contraption. (Due to the way the streets around here are laid out, it's difficult not to pass that house when coming or going from ours.) *Do those people know your life has turned into A Nightmare on Elm Street? Because their set design is awfully appropriate.* She gives me a nudge in the ribs as I turn away from the window: *Sheesh, just look at that thing! Too funny, eh?*

I don't respond. For the past 56 minutes I've complied with Sane Me's instructions to sit in the big armchair and do needlepoint ... to eat a deli turkey slice straight out of the package while standing before the refrigerator ... to wash dishes ... to go around back outside and make another careful study of the wrought-iron fence above the stairwell (*gotta admit it's a nice drop; stupid thorny rose bush*)

Fury said to
  a mouse, That

he met
in the
house,
'Let us
both go to law:
I will
prosecute
you.

to sit in the big armchair coloring with the colored pencils in the coloring book … to pace up and down on the flagstones of the front garden humming "I'm Looking Over a Four-Leaf Clover" … to eat a piece of cheese and a graham cracker … finally to stand in the living room, swaying gently side to side, riding the boat deck, looking but not looking at the devil down the block. Matt is in the basement office, working or perhaps napping; in the silences between the howls of Animatronic Lucifer, I think I can hear light snores. Then my phone buzzes; it's a text message from CVS to "pick up Rx QUE." I don my coat and scarf and head off again.

Earlier, on my late morning walk, I had a call with Dr. Funar. She asked me how I was doing. "Not good," I said, crying a little. "Not good. The anxiety is so bad." I turned the corner onto Galisteo, phone pressed to my ear, wiping my dripping nose with a gloved hand.

"Any side effects from the Zoloft?"

"No … I mean, I don't know. I have a sore throat. My whole head is itching. The vertigo is worse, everything is getting worse, and I don't know, I just feel so terrible all the time."

"How is the Ambien working?"

"It works for maybe three hours. I tried taking a hydroxyzine when I wake up in the night, but it doesn't seem to help. Isn't there anything, anything else for sleep?"

"Yes, let's try Seroquel."

Into my mind swims the wistful moonlit face of the fawn girl wrapped in her light blue blanket, sitting on the scrubby ground against the coyote fence out behind Unity, chatting with me as we wait for our meds. *Seroquel is the best ... It's the only thing that works for me.*

"Oh, OK, yes. Seroquel. Is it OK to take it with Ambien?"

"Yes, it's fine. You can break it in half if you want. Quetiapine is the generic name."

"OK." Crying a little harder. "Are you sending it in right now?"

"Yes, yes, right now." Her voice is kind, reassuring as ever.

At two-thirty I get the text message from CVS saying it's ready. Now I'm walking down Galisteo, turning right on Lomita then up Don Diego, across the parking lot (*put on your mask, it's in your coat pocket*) into the store, where I feign normality (*but honestly, girl, how much longer can we keep this up?*) as I interact with the pharmacy cashier, but he must have pressed the secret druggie-alert button or something because the pharmacist comes over and says to me with furrowed brow: "Hi, Ms. Davis. Are you aware of the possible interactions between quetiapine and Ambien? They can be a little dangerous."

Come, I'll
take no
denial:
We must
have a
trial;

"Um ... oh, um, well, I guess my psychiatrist is aware. She said it was all right."

His face clears. "Oh, good, you're under a psychiatrist's care? No problem, then. Sorry."

"Ha-ha, it's fine."

"Just needed to check."

"Yes, thanks, of course, thanks."

"Bye, now."

"Bye."

I leave the store and walk along Cordova to the rose park, wander around and into the park, sit down on a low stone wall. I pull out my phone, type "quetiapine" into Google, then with left hand pocketed against the cold and right hand grasping my phone (*just like the Mock Turtle*) start scrolling through drug information. Quetiapine is an antipsychotic which, I read, "at lower doses has a sedative effect." *Mm-hmm ... heard that one before, haven't we?* I switch to a drug review site

> For
> really
> this
> morning
> I've
> nothing
> to do.'

where the reviews are mostly positive, ratings in the 6.0 – 7.5 range, *so that's good, maybe this will really be it, maybe blue blanket fawn girl was right and this one really will do the trick.* Other websites mention the perils of mixing quetiapine with benzo derivatives, such as Ambien, but, *pish, at this point does it even matter?* Next I search out Zoloft reviews and scan those, *girl, you've looked up Zoloft how many times?* noting once again how everyone agrees that "it gets worse before it gets better," *see, you just have to hang on.* The toddler's whine is getting loud now, so I rise and continue on my way, walking back up Galisteo, right on Coronado, now I'm praying—for some reason the afternoon walks are devoted to prayer more than tree assessment—crying again, *Hail Mary full of grace the Lord is with thee, Blessed art thou among women and blessed is* … wiping my nose with one hand, clutching the CVS brown paper bag with the other, walking faster, now praying out loud: "God DAMN it I don't care if I never sleep again I will NOT let this beat me, do you hear me, God? I will NOT kill myself, for Emily's sake, I will hang on for her sake" *that's right it's not about you, not about you, she'll be destroyed if you kill yourself, and the Seroquel is going to help, it's going to let you sleep, fawn girl said so.*

My aching legs and the sinking sun are demanding that I head home. My steps slow as I walk along Booth, left on Granada, up the gravel driveway to the kitchen door. As I enter the tiny mudroom and take off my scarf and coat, breathing in the fusty indoor smell, a leaden crush of despair sweeps through me: Home now. Stale deadness. Nothing to do. Nowhere to go. And tomorrow—tomorrow the clocks fall back for daylight saving, which means waking up at 2:47 not 3:47, and there's going to be nine inches of snow and that *thing* down the street, groaning and glaring at me. How, how am I going to make it through tomorrow? *Somehow. Somehow. The Seroquel might work, yes it might, wait and see.*

One indoor game I can still play is called Packing for the Hospital. On Emily's quilted twin bed (in her room which is now my sitting room, as Matt calls it, making me think of that story "The Yellow Wallpaper" with the crazy woman who creeps round and round with her shoulder to the wall) is a neat array of insanity supplies: notebooks, needlepoint, coloring book and pencils, crossword puzzles, water bottle, medical file folder, origami kit, wallet, Post-its with key phone numbers. Also my backpack and purse, which are the packing game's focus. Quietly, quietly, so Matt won't hear, I pack, unpack, and repack the bags with a morphing set of clothing, toiletries, and selections from the insanity supplies. While I'm playing this game I'm thinking

Said the

mouse to

the cur,

'Such a

trial,

dear sir,

shouldn't I go to the hospital? I mean it's like a 35-minute walk, that's not so far really, I can just take off early in the morning and not even tell Matt, he doesn't need to know, I can check myself in, I'm an adult, how many pairs of underwear will I need? I guess it all depends on how long they keep me, but Dr. Funar and Dr. Ortega said don't go, Matt says they just keep the students on a 48-hour hold then kick them out on the street and anyway there's Covid, we're not supposed to take up beds during this time of Covid, you can't go, forget it, unpack everything and put it back and stop being so ridiculous! But look, Matt can't take this much longer, I *have* to go. I'd better slim down this bag of toiletries ... really, do I need moisturizer? No you don't, take that out, but better pack both pairs of glasses, the old and the new, put them both in the side pockets, that's it, but not the Kindle, you can't even read anymore so why do you need a Kindle, oh and what about tights, I'd better pack a spare pair of tights because that way if I do decide to kill myself I'll have the means handy, all right now tiptoe to the linen closet, get the big baggie of meds, don't let Matt hear, put that in the backpack, good, it just fits ... forget the needlepoint, you won't be able to fool the hospital people the way you did CT Lenora

With no

jury or

judge,

would be

wasting

our breath.'

but tomorrow there will be snow, you can't walk all the way in the snow, in the dark, c'mon man, and what if someone tries to rob me or kill me or something, well who cares if they kill you but if they steal your stuff you're going to be seriously upset so just think about that

    wasting
     our breath.'

until six o'clock. Dinnertime now and I'm sitting in the big shabby armchair in my sitting room, forcing down a dish of mac and cheese with tuna and peas prepared by Matt. I'm wearing my old fleecy black hat in a vain attempt to muffle the ear-piercing clangs as he stirs his own helping on the stovetop; my back is wedged between cushions in a vain attempt to stop the ground's pitching; my throat hurts, my scalp hurts, my bones hurt. No trick or treaters, at least; thank God for the pandemic. In a few minutes I will find an episode of the Great British Baking Show Masterclass on Netflix and set it to play on my laptop, Paul Hollywood and Mary Whatsername chatting expertly about sticky toffee pudding as I sit wedged in the armchair coloring, coloring, in a vain attempt to take my brain away from the danger while still letting it be on guard as it wants to be ... no, it wants more than that ... it wants to be

     'I'll be
      judge,
     I'll be
      jury,'
   Said

judge and jury, interrogator and warden, prisoner and executioner, all housed together forever in the red groaning panopticon, where eyes never close and torment never stops

> cunning
> old Fury;

but at last I move on to the jigsaw puzzle, saved for mid-eve-
ning because it's the only thing I can really spend hours on at a
stretch: three hundred pieces, a nighttime holiday scene of a fine
old steam train pulled up to a station in the snow, heavy snow,
starry sky, a Model T Ford with snow on the fenders, a woman in
1940s coat and hat walking from the tracks toward the car with
a beribboned box in her arms, evergreen wreaths with pretty red
bows in the station windows, the engine lamps shining warm
gold on the snow but the train itself looming, menacing, a great
black iron beast in the Christmas dark, and I'm staring at the
puzzle pieces laid out on the white poster board, I find one, fit it
in, cast a sideways glance at the mirror on the closet door to see

> cunning
> old Fury;
> 'I'll try
> the whole
> cause,

a very thin, almost emaciated woman with messy gray hair, hag-
gard gray face, and an alarmingly hunched back, leaning over a
table. I look away from the woman, repulsed, and a very clear
voice in my head says: *It is not possible to feel this bad and still be
alive*

yet you are alive, you *are* alive, and Matt says, "Did you take
a hydroxyzine?" "Dr. Ortega said only as needed." "I don't care,
take one, take one right now." "Fine, I will, fine," cut the round
white pill in half and swallow, soon the world goes out of focus

far away so slow so tired oh my god so tired but Security Brain says *NO SLEEP!* so get up and walk around, walk around the living room, keep walking until it wears off, which it does in half an hour and then it's the puzzle again for another two hours and finally it's eleven-thirty time to get ready for bed brush teeth floss teeth gargle with salt water throat is so sore ow owwww have a pee owwww that hurts too no UTI please no UTI get into pajamas get the Ambien Tylenol Hydroxyzine Seroquel put them in the bowl get the glass of water put it on the bedside table turn on the electric radiator get in bed try to read a book it's no use no use Matt comes to ask do you need anything Bear, No thanks, no, just about to take the meds, at a quarter past midnight swallow the Ambien Tylenol Seroquel and you know right then for absolute certain that the Seroquel isn't going to do one damn thing and you will wake up at 2:47 to the storm waters rising and the wolf-jailer cackling but oh well lights out remember you'll still have your trees and at a quarter to one just before the suffocating black velvet coma curtain descends the sleet starts to patter on the window making you aware that tomorrow (arriving in moments, lasting forever) will be worse, and the next day even worse, and down, down, down you'll go because there is no bottom to this panopticon and winter is coming and the verdict is certain, cunning old Fury, judge and jury, will try the whole cause

>   and
>   condemn
>   you
>   to
>   death.

I made it three more days. The blizzard fell thick and wet, and the snow hung around covering my walk routes in dirty impass-able heaps. On Tuesday, I decided I must be in actual Hell.

On Wednesday, November the fourth, at 6:15 a.m. Mountain Standard Time, I pull on my boots, zip up my coat, wind my lavender scarf around my neck, set my old fleecy hat on my head, take several steps across the kitchen, then—sit down on the floor. I have done all the running I can do, and there is, all at once, nothing left: no intellect, no will, no emotion, nothing. Just a soft gauzy fall of nonbeing where the person formerly known as Jocelyn used to be.

Matt ascends the basement stairs. "What're you doing, Bear?"

A scratchy whisper: "Hospital, hospital, hospital."

Thirteen hours later I am being pushed in a wheelchair down the bright echoing corridors of St. Giles, to the psych ward.

PART III

DOWN
THE
RABBIT
HOLE

CHAPTER 8

POOL OF TEARS

R ight after I was trundled through the big white door into the small dim room with the round table flanked by the two nurses and heard the latch click behind me, I suffered a brief but total meltdown in which I flung out a hand toward an oblong of light, which I sensed was the portal to a larger space (the room with the promised mountain view?), and shrieked: "We're going in there, right?! We're not staying in here!! We're going in there, right?!" Had this been Orwell's Room 101, I would have been screaming *Do it to Julia, not to me! Do it to Julia!*

Nurse A—white-skinned, older, with crinkly eyes and an oatmeal-colored bob—smiled serenely. "Yes, yes, we'll be going in there soon." Lifting my bundled belongings off my lap, she handed them to Nurse B—brown-skinned, younger, with chunky glasses and slick pixie cut—who did something to make them disappear while I clutched the wheelchair arms, convulsing. Then Nurse A seemed to realize what had me so perturbed. "Oh! No, no," she said with a jolly laugh, "this isn't your *room!* This is just where we do your checkup. Won't take long."

I subsided, still shaking. Sane Me had resumed her position up above and behind my right shoulder, from which vantage point she was eying the two nurses with critical interest, noticing the narrow lockers arrayed along one wall, guessing that this space must be a staffroom of some kind—but not saying anything as yet. Probably she knew I wouldn't have heard her.

"I'm Nurse [*noises*]," said Nurse A.

"I'm Nurse [*different noises*]," said Nurse B, next to whom had appeared a rolling cart laden with medical devices, which she proceeded to push around to my left side, maneuvering deftly the tight space between wheelchair and wall while remarking, "I'm just going to take your blood pressure." Obedient, mindful that whatever I did I *must not* anger my captors, I held out a trembling arm for the cuff. Tears ran down my cheeks, snot down my lips and chin. My lungs heaved, gulping at the disinfected air. Was I still wearing a mask? I don't remember.

"So, how would you rate your anxiety level right now?" asked Nurse A, as if asking how I'd rate the service on my Hyundai. "On a scale of one to ten?"

"Ten!" [*sniff, sob, gasp*]

"Yeah." Nodding, she made a note on a clipboard. "I would have said ten."

Way down under the layers of fear and phlegm, like the princess's pea under her stack of mattresses, I felt a hard pellet of satisfaction that my top rating had been accepted so readily.

My blood pressure and pulse oxygen were noted. My temperature was taken. A stethoscope was pressed to my back and chest. A scale was indicated, I stood on it, and my weight was recorded. My scalp, neck, and forearms were inspected. I continued to sob throughout, and the two nurses maintained a tone much like that of the ER staffers who had rallied round the drunken Carpenter a few hours ago: brisk, unruffled, polite but in command.

"Now," said Nurse A, "we're just going to check your body for wounds."

(Wounds? Like needle marks? Or cut marks? I don't have those. Do I? *Do* I??)

"Let's first have you stand up and take off your shirt and sweater." I stood with jelly legs and removed my upper garments, leaving my bra in place. Nurse B went around behind me and looked at my back while Nurse A looked at my front. Then Nurse A produced a medium-sized white towel, like the towels you get in hotels, stretched it out in front of me like a screen, except it wasn't actually screening anything, and said, "Now if you could just lift up your bra real quick." I did, and she looked at my exposed chest over the top of the towel. "OK, good. Now if you'd sit back down and take off your shoes and your jeans."

I sat back down in the wheelchair. I must have started crying harder because Nurse B said firmly, "It's all right. This is a safe place." (Is it? I don't believe you)

As I bent to take off my shoes, Nurse A added: "This is the worst part. It gets better after this." (Does it? I don't believe you)

I removed my black sneakers and handed them over. Nurse A received them with a small frown: "Oh, dear, these have laces. I'm afraid you can't have shoes with laces."

(Oh God no they're going to take away my shoes noooo)

"No! [*sob*] I have ver- [*gulp*] vertigo. I need shoes to help me balance. I *need* them!"

Nurse A seemed sympathetic. "Well, we can take the laces off, if you like, and you can wear them like slippers. How's that?"

"OK. Yes, yes, go ahead. Take the laces off [*sniff, gurgle*] please. Thank you."

"I'll do it in a minute." She put the shoes on the round table. "Now if you could take off your jeans." I did, fumbling with button and zipper, slithering out of them while still seated.

"Oh … you're wearing pantyhose!" Nurse A seemed quite shocked.

I looked down at my waist. I had forgotten all about the pantyhose. (Are pantyhose bad?! I'm sorry. I'm sorry. Don't be mad at me, please don't be mad at me! Oh God what is happening why did I come here this is the end I'm going to die I'm never getting out God help me God help me Hail Mary full of grace Hail Mary full of grace Hail Mary *Relax, dingbat* wait what?)

I said, Relax, dingbat.

Mad Me: What? What? Who's that?

Sane Me: *It's me, silly. They can't let you have pantyhose. Pantyhose are like shoelaces: ligatures, right? You really thought these folks wouldn't see through your nutso scheme?*

Mad Me: Jesus! [*cough*] Where have you been?! How was I to know pantyhose weren't allowed? No one told me! Anyway [*sniffle*] I only put them on for warmth!

Sane Me: *Uh-huh. Warmth. Surrre ya did.*

Mad Me: What do you m—God, I hate you! I hate you!! I've never been so scared in my life, and you can't even be nice to me! Go away!!

Sane Me: *Sheesh. Just trying to help.*

Mad Me: Fine! Fine [*cough*]. At least you're speaking to me again. Thanks a bunch.

Sane Me: *You're welcome. So now, let's try to focus. This is a safe place, you know.*

This entire exchange unfolded in half a second and was heard, naturally, by me alone. It was accompanied by a gentle *boing*—the sound, maybe, of a psyche hitting rock bottom and being yanked ever so slightly upward.

"… afraid you can't have pantyhose here," Nurse A was saying with a smile. "It's a shame, really; I've always liked them. Not many people wear them these days. I like how they hold you in; you feel contained." She patted her belly and looked at Nurse B, who murmured agreement.

"Yes," I said, patting my own belly. "Contained. Ha-ha."

She had me take them off and stand for an inspection of my legs and feet. Then she stretched out the white towel again, saying, "Now just take down your underwear real quick for me." I complied, and she peered over the terrycloth screen at my pelvis while Nurse B checked my rear.

Sane Me: *God, this towel business is ridiculous, eh?*

Mad Me: I guess. But [*sniffle*] I dunno, isn't it also kind of ... humane?

Sane Me: *Jesus, what now, Stockholm syndrome? Well, whatever works for you.*

While I put my clothes back on, sans pantyhose, Nurse B rolled away the vitals cart and Nurse A plucked and tugged the laces from my sneakers. It took her a while; she remarked on the difficulty as I sat wiping my eyes and nose on my sweater sleeve. At length she finished and gave the shoes back. "Is that going to work?" she asked as I stood up and took a few tentative steps, watching the black laceless tongues protruding floppily from the tops of my feet.

"Yes, that's perfect," I said. "Thank you."

"Of course. OK, here we go."

Shuffling, as through a pool of tears, I followed her through the lighted doorway.

————

There might have been a mountain view beyond the windows of the dayroom, but since it was nighttime there was nothing to see but blurry reflections swimming on an inky void covered by steel mesh. The room itself was a rectangle, maybe forty feet by twenty. Along the left wall under the windows ran a row of cabinets topped by a Formica counter; along the right wall, four doors to bedrooms stood open. At the far end, a long table stretched in front of more cabinets, a bookcase, and another bedroom door. Behind me, a glass-fronted nurses' station kept eyes on the whole space, panopticon-style. The furniture comprised a dozen wooden armchairs and couches plus several oblong coffee tables and round tea tables, all neatly arranged on the clean linoleum floor and all with the look of a college dorm circa 1985: sturdy yet comfortable, with vinyl cushions in blue and brown. Fixed high on the wall between two of the bedroom doors was a flat-screen TV. The volume was cranked up loud. I had the impression of four, maybe five people sitting in various spots. The room itself was far from horrible, but the steel-meshed windows looming darkly down the left wall created a sense of being at the bottom of the sea.

Nurse A—whose name, Annette, had by now osmosed into my brain—showed me to my bedroom, the second one in the row. It was pretty bleak. Sticking out from one wall were two twin beds with dark-gray cotton blankets (*oh look, the legs are bolted to the floor; guess they're onto that trachea-crushing gambit, eh?*) plus two low bedside tables. Along the other wall was a credenza with a few shelves and drawers underneath, plus two wooden chairs. Fluorescent ceiling lights buzzed softly; heavily bolted and barred windows looked out onto nothing. No rugs, no lamps, no drapes, no closet, no color. Immediately to the left as you walked in, screened only by a white vinyl curtain, was a bathroom; it contained a small stainless-steel sink with no mirror, a big stainless-steel toilet (*prison vibes, but hey at least it has a seat*), a tiny white shower stall, and two stainless-steel towel bars mounted flush to the wall, rendering them useless for hanging towels—or anything else, presumably.

Would they even give me towels? I wondered. Following Nurse Annette back out to the dayroom, I noticed one stuffed under the bedroom door. I nudged it with my toe.

"Yeah, so," she said with a shrug and a chuckle, "we require these doors to be open at all times, but you don't have to keep it open *all* the way, just so long as it's never closed. But this door is sort of broken, it wants to swing all the way open, so someone put a towel under to keep it halfway closed. Sorry about that ..."

I stared at her, struggling to follow. Who had put the towel there? Was it an official towel? Was I allowed to move it? If I moved it and closed (or opened) the door, what would happen? Nothing, probably; then again, who knew what the rules were, here in the real panopticon. If Nurse Annette had said towels were to be used only as nudity screens and doorstops, and that the punishment for a closed (or open) door was electric shocks, I would have believed her.

"... in the middle of a shift change, so it will be a little while before we can inventory your things. We'll get to it just as soon as we can. And I'll get you some toiletries, in a bit. For now, I'll let you relax." She walked off to the glass-fronted fishbowl enclosure, swiped her ID card, and joined the four other nurses who were sitting within on swivel chairs, having a meeting. Piled on a table behind them I could see my purse, backpack, and Elephant.

"Let you relax"? Yeah, right. The wolf-jailer was back, but instead of a whip he had a box that he was trying to stuff me into. Claustrophobia squeezed my gut as I looked around the dayroom with its locked doors, locked windows, and absolute impossibility of escape. I knew they couldn't legally keep me as long as I wasn't a danger to myself or others; clearly, though, there would be no getting out tonight. Panic started to bubble, but, *Hey! Hey! You chose this,* barked Sane Me. *You're choosing this. Breathe. Walk.* I began to pace up and down, quite fast, in front of the nurses' fishbowl: Ten paces toward the windows. U-turn. Ten paces away from the windows. U-turn. Ten paces toward ... Flap-flap went my laceless shoes. Every time I faced the windows I could see my reflection wavering against the black void outside. *Keep walking. It's a room like any other room. Walk, walk, you'll be all right, walk, walk, you'll be all right.*

As I paced, I began to register, fuzzily, the other patients. On the couch right in front of the TV, watching it with seeming enjoyment, were a muscular man with a bandana around his bald head and a petite woman with long dark curly hair; on a chair behind them, also watching the TV, was a big mustachioed man with his cast-encased right foot propped on a coffee table. Sitting at a round tea table in the corner farthest from me, a little in the shadows, was a woman with long wavy brown hair who was coloring or drawing something. Standing at the near end of the counter, back to the room, was a man of slight build, dark hair, working intently on a jigsaw puzzle. All wore regular street clothes. All looked much younger than I.

Then there was Julia Roberts: teeth bared in her trademark grin, hands full of shopping bags, snazzy white hat and dress turning the heads of passersby, prancing down Rodeo Drive to "PRETTY WOMAN, WALKIN DOWN THE STREET, PRETTY WOMAN, THE KIND I'D LIKE TO MEET ..." There was a shred of comfort in the realization that even here, in Madland, the same damn movies were on every damn night; on the other hand, the music was loud, painfully loud, and as I paced I pressed my fingers to my ears, wondering if the television stayed on 24-7, as in an airport. It seemed unlikely, but again, how was I to know?

Everyone so far was ignoring me, thank goodness. The nurses went on with their meeting and the five inmates went on with their activities as I paced up and down, trying to be invisible and periodically blocking my ears against the shrilling noise of the TV. I had just decided that the folks here looked relatively normal and, more important, weren't going to accost me, when, just as I reached the end of a downward lap, the bald bandana man on the couch twisted round, thrust out a silver object, and shouted: "Do ya wanna use the *phone*?!"

I stopped dead, horrified, shaking my head "no," feeling my face pull into a rictus of fear and misery, silently willing this maniac to leave me alone. I turned on my heel and headed back toward the windows (He's mad as a hatter, mad as a hatter, mad as … If he attacks me, what will I do, where will I run, will the nurses help? oh God), but when I reached the end of the lap and pivoted, he was facing the TV again, watching Richard Gere snap the jewelry case puckishly on the fingers of a begowned, laughing Julia Roberts. I looked over at the nurses. They either hadn't noticed the phone assault or didn't think it worth noticing.

I kept a sharp eye on the Mad Hatter as I continued to pace.

Some minutes later, the brown-haired girl coloring in the back corner accidentally knocked a nerf ball off her table. It bounced and rolled toward me, coming to a stop near my feet. I looked at it for a moment, then, mustering my courage, bent down, grasped it, and rolled it back to her. She bent down to catch it and said quietly, "Thanks."

"You're welcome."

See, they're not going to attack you. She's not, anyway. Dunno about the Mad Hatter.

I broke away from my up-and-down track and struck out for the Formica counter under the windows. Inching along, careful to make no noise, I came upon some boxed jigsaw puzzles. With surreptitious glances at Jigsaw Guy, who was making progress on his puzzle and clearly couldn't have cared less what I was doing, I opened a box with a picture of a cardinal on a snow-covered branch, dumped out a few of the 500 pieces, touched one or two, and abandoned that idea at once. Moving on down the counter I found a black plastic file holder stocked with coloring pages, most with Christian themes: stained-glass windows, haloed angels, saints. A couple of bins of worn crayons and felt markers sat nearby, smelling of wax and acetone. I sidled around Coloring Girl's table, averted my eyes from the open bedroom door on the far wall, and approached the bookcase. Here was a large collection of tattered magazines and a much smaller collection of books representing a variety of genres: novels, self-help, spirituality, poetry. My eyes fell on a book with a gray and orange cover: *Fierce Conversations,* by Susan Scott. I knew that book! I knew it from my corporate training days. I had read it. I knew it. A ripple of assurance, barely perceptible, passed through the pool of tears as I pulled out the book, hugged it to my chest, and shuffled back to the nurses' station. I knocked on the glass.

A nurse whizzed over on her swivel chair and slid the window open. "Yes?"

"I'm ... sorry, I'm just wondering when I'm going to get my ... my clothes and stuff?"

"Soon. We're just in the middle of a shift change. Very soon."

"Thing is, I'd really like my stuffed elephant. Do you think I could have my elephant?"

"We're getting to it just as quickly as we can."

"Oh, OK. Thanks." The window slid shut.

I paced some more, clutching My Book tightly. Then, suddenly re-noticing the white towel jammed under my bedroom door, and seized by the sense that such an arrangement was ineffective and unsanitary, not to mention ugly, I set off across the dayroom for a second time, to the bookshelf, where I selected the heaviest tome there—something about investing—carried it back to the door, and kicked aside the towel, all the while side-eyeing the nurses to see if any of them was going to yell at me for misusing the reading material. None did. For the next ten minutes I occupied myself with placing the tome at various spots on the floor, adjusting the door to various states of openness, and checking to see if the gap was wide enough for me to traverse but not wide enough for an audience to see inside. The door was heavy and did seem to want to swing open, but eventually I found the point where the book held it suitably ajar. Meanwhile the nurses and my fellow patients paid no attention, and gradually it dawned on me that I had come to a place where crazy was the norm, indeed, crazy was *expected,* therefore nobody would be irritated if I obsessed over the door, nobody would frown and tell me to stop fiddling. *So long as you're not causing real trouble,* said Sane Me, *no one cares. Isn't that nice? No one cares.*

After a while Nurse Annette emerged from the glass enclosure and handed me a few towels and a white paper bag, which I took to my room to inspect. The bag contained: toothbrush, toothpaste, mouthwash, deodorant, lotion, and bottle of combined shampoo-bodywash, all travel sized, plus a small black comb and a pair of grippy socks, light blue with a smiley-face design.* I set about arranging and rearranging these items: most should go in the bathroom, obviously, but maybe the comb should go by the bed and socks on the credenza shelf? No soap ledge in the shower, so where should the shampoo-bodywash go? On the floor, I guess. The stuck-to-the-wall towel bars were useless, so I laid the towels on the recessed shelf next to the sink. Returning to the bedroom, I removed my watch—which Nurse No-Name, upstairs at Intake, had said I could keep, though warning me the hospital wasn't liable were it to be stolen—and arranged it next to My Comb and My Book on the bedside table. I put the empty white paper bag neatly on its side at the end of the credenza. Finally, and with some trepidation, I took the pillow off the other twin bed and put it atop my own. *Sorry, bitches, it's medically necessary.*

Yet another interesting challenge presented itself when Nurse Priya (that was the name of Nurse B) brought me another paper bag, this one holding my contact lens case and saline solution. After placing case and solution on the bathroom sink and laying Bag No. 2 next to Bag No. 1, I turned my mind to how I was going to insert and remove my contacts without the aid of

---

* Years later, I would learn that mental hospital stays are known to the in-crowd as "grippy sock vacations." I'm proud to say I still have my pair, tucked safely in my pajama drawer. Actually, two pairs; the story of the second pair is still to come.

a mirror. I didn't want to wear my glasses all day; the ear stems hurt my head. After a minute or two of prowling around the bedroom in the vague hope a mirror would appear, I realized one of the windows might do: the heavy shade could be pushed up— no cords, of course—and the break-proof glass, covered on the outside in steel mesh, made a reflective surface over the darkness. I bent down, peered at my own face (*hmm, hardly a sharp image, but it'll do, it'll do*), then cupped my hands like horse blinkers and gazed through. I couldn't quite tell, but there seemed to be a small courtyard or air shaft out there, which meant that the morning light outside might still be dim enough to make the window a serviceable looking glass, albeit one impossible to pass through. *See, there are virtues to everything,* said Sane Me, *even a room without a view.* I felt proud of my ingenuity.

"Hi, Jocelyn," said the young blonde nurse in royal-blue scrubs. "Would you mind if we talk for a little bit, over here at the desk?"

"Sure," I said. I was in a marginally calmer state. At around 7:45 they'd started my inventory; Nurse Annette had called me over to ask whether she could cut the drawstring off my pajama pants, to which I said yes go ahead, thinking they'd probably sag off my hips but better saggy pajamas than no pajamas. Upon handing me the stack of approved clothing (topped by Elephant, thank goodness), she explained I couldn't have anything else I'd brought—not my Kindle, not my phone, not the colored pencils, not the toiletries, and certainly not the notebook and crossword books with the sharp spiral-wire bindings, because *you'd be surprised,* the Mock Turtle had said—"but this one is OK," and she handed over the slim brown stapled notebook from the True Healing Center, in which I'd recorded my doctors' phone numbers and medication notes. *Okeydokey, then. At least you've got one notebook.* Now it was about 8:15. Just over an hour had passed since I'd arrived in the ward, though it seemed much longer. I was pacing again, both Elephant and My Book clutched to my chest, when the blonde nurse approached and asked if we could talk. I followed her over to the desk in front of the fishbowl.

"I'm Nurse Wendy," she said as we sat down. "Is it OK if I ask you some questions?" Nodding assent, I placed My Book and Elephant in my lap, grabbed a tissue to wipe my nose, and thought: She seems nice. Her youth—she couldn't have been out of her twenties—short stature, round face, cheerful demeanor, and wavy blonde bob gave her something of the air of a 1940s Hollywood starlet, a girl-next-door type who'd be cast in ingénue roles.

She started down a list of questions printed on a form, noting my answers for me. She asked about my symptoms; about my employment, housing situation, family situation, and education; drug use, sexual abuse, and domestic abuse ("none"); sleep and appetite ("terrible"); suicidal ideation ("lots"). I liked that she wasn't staring at a computer and that I could see what she was writing. I liked that she didn't dispute any of my answers— she nodded and smiled through her mask at each—and that she seemed mildly impressed by my two master's degrees.

"Next is a question about your goals while you're here. We ask you to set goals for eating and sleeping. What would you say for eating?"

"Sorry, what? *Goals* for eating?"

She tilted her head disarmingly. "Ha-ha, yes, like, what percentage of each meal would you like to eat?"

"Oh." I suddenly realized I was hungry. I pushed the thought away. "I guess … all of it?"

"OK, great!" She beamed and circled *100%* on the form.

Then I recalled the oatmeal raisin cookie that had come with the Salisbury steak. What if such a cookie came with every meal? Would they make me eat it, now that I'd promised to?

"But I'm not going to eat any desserts! I'm not going to eat any cookies, or, or … cake!"

"That's totally fine," said Nurse Wendy, with a wave of her pen. "Now, in terms of a goal for sleep, what would you say? How many hours a night?"

As I'd given up weeks ago the hope of ever sleeping normally again, this question seemed meaningless, almost mocking.

"Um … you mean a *realistic* goal? Or how much I *want* to sleep?"

"It's up to you." She laughed, pleasantly. "I mean, you might as well say what you want."

Might I? I guess I might. I drew a deep breath. "Well, I don't know … I suppose I'd *like* to get, let's say, sev—" At the last second, I chickened out. "Six hours."

"Great!" She wrote it down, *6 hrs.*

There was a rumbling noise. I looked up to see a cart with foodstuffs on it: bags of chips, pudding cups, apples, juice cups. The cart-pushing nurse left it by the desk and withdrew.

"Oh! There are snacks!"

"What? Oh, yes," said Nurse Wendy, turning to look. "We bring in the snack cart in the morning, afternoon, and evening. It's mostly chips and stuff, but there's always fruit."

Relief swept my brain. Plans to stash emergency food supplies in my room took shape.

We moved on to the topic of medications. I told her what I took at bedtime: acyclovir, progesterone, Ambien. She said the acyclovir and progesterone were fine, they had those, but she'd need to check with the on-call doctor about the Ambien. She asked permission to take my vitals—blood pressure, temperature, pulse ox—then produced a large clear plastic water cup with a lid and straw, said I could keep it, and asked if I'd like her to fill it. "Yes please," I said, thought about specifying "No ice," thought that might be perceived as too demanding (*the flight attendants are here primarily for your safety*) and watched her go to a door to the left of the heavily alarmed main entrance, swipe her card, and enter. While she was gone, I took the opportunity to inspect the snack cart. I selected a Red Delicious apple and a foil-topped cup of cranberry juice.

Nurse Wendy returned with the filled water container. "I gave you just a little ice," she said. "I didn't know if you wanted it with or without."

"Oh," I said. "Thanks. I prefer no ice. But this is fine. Thanks! Thank you so much."

"Of course," she said, smiling sweetly. "I'll check with the doctor about the Ambien."

I took my snacks, sat down as far as possible from the other inmates, ate the apple, and pretended to watch the end of *Pretty Woman* while pondering where to hide the cranberry juice cup. The movie over, I went to my room and tiptoed around assessing various spots, finally settling on the credenza shelf behind my folded red sweatshirt. I wondered what they'd do if they caught me, but I figured the no-food-in-bedrooms rule was more about sanitation than self-harm—after all, not even the Mock Turtle's clever nephew could kill himself with a juice cup—so the punishment for stashing unopened food surely wouldn't be severe. Besides, I thought, as long as I didn't give them cause, they were unlikely to ransack my room, for such an invasion would be at odds with the courteous ethos which, I was realizing, prevailed among the wardens of Madland, with their towel screens, evening snack carts, and inquiries as to ice preferences. I returned to the dayroom feeling good about having added My Juice to my limited stash of possessions, if only for tonight.

Batshit you are, laughed Sane Me. *100 percent batshit.*

Soon Nurse Wendy reappeared. "Hi, Jocelyn. I asked the doctor in charge about the Ambien, and she said we don't have the extended-release kind, but I can give you the regular kind, the five milligrams."

"Not the ten milligrams? I've been taking the bigger dose. Dr. Funar prescribed it."

She shook her head with apparently genuine regret. "No, I'm really sorry, she said only the five milligrams."

Why can't they ever dispense the Ambien right? "Well, OK, but if that's all I get, I'm gonna be awake at 1:30." My voice rose to an anxious squeak. "I'll be freaking out. I'm telling you!"

"I understand. And when you wake up, I can give you some Ativan if you want. I'll be right here, all night. I'm the nurse assigned to you, and I'm going to look after you."

I stared at her, processing the "when you wake up" (so she believes me), the "Ativan if you want" (so she can give me other drugs, real drugs, not the Ambien though, weird) and the "I'm assigned to you, I'm going to look after you" (so she's my nurse, my person, and she'll be right here all night, for me. That sounds good)

"OK," I said. "That sounds good."

"Great," she said. "Do you want to take your meds now?"

"Oh." I looked at the clock: nine-thirty. "Could I maybe take them at, like, ten-thirty?"

"Yes, absolutely."

I changed into my pajamas—the lack of drawstrings had the waistband loose but not fatally so—then joined Coloring Girl at the table in the back corner. She introduced herself as Lindsey. "Jocelyn," I replied. We didn't talk, just sat and colored until ten o'clock arrived, whereupon the TV was switched off and there was a general move toward the bedrooms.

I decided to take a shower. The faucet in the tiny stall required immense strength to turn on, but once on, the water was unexpectedly hot, the pressure impressively strong. Afterward I laid the damp towel across the no-hanging towel bar, resumed my pajamas, brushed my teeth, and got into bed. I tried to read My Book, but the thicket of words resisted comprehension as usual, so I just stared at page one until Nurse Wendy arrived with my meds in a doll-sized paper cup. There was a high-tech system: for each pill, she first used a device to scan the barcode on my wristband, then scanned the code on the pill package, tore open the package, and dropped the pill in the paper cup. Once everything was scanned, she handed me the cup and watched as I swallowed the pills, one by one, chasing them with the water from my strawed water container. She explained they'd be checking on me every fifteen minutes throughout the night.

"What? Every fifteen *minutes*?"

"Yes. We try hard not to wake you. But we do use a flashlight. Just so you know."

Wow. Those healing center folks with their "every two hours." Amateurs!

The ward had grown quiet. The bedroom was cool, almost cold; I had tried, earlier, to turn up the thermostat, but the heat didn't seem to be working, so I'd pulled the gray cotton blanket off the other bed and heaped it onto mine. I figured I'd already stolen the pillow, so why not? Nurse Wendy did not remark on blankets or pillows but gathered up the empty pill packs and her barcode scanner and wished me good night. Standing in the doorway, she asked if I'd like her to turn off the light.

"I'm going to read a little longer. Is that OK? To leave the light on, I mean?"

"Yes, of course! Would you like your water filled up?"

"Yes, please."

"No ice, right?"

"Right. Thank you so much."

Later, I lay on my back in the semidarkness, the light from the dayroom fluorescing dully in the half-open doorway, my head propped high on my possibly illicit pillows, listening to the slow drip of the shower faucet I'd been unable to turn off completely, feeling the mattress undulating as I waited for the Ambien to kick in. The two empty white paper bags on the credenza were floating up and down like two small, square, luminous ghosts; this was a new phenomenon, which I found quite soothing. *You're hallucinating*, said Sane Me. Whatever, said

Mad Me; it's comfortable here. Anyway, I'm sick of you trying to control every little thing. Look at the paper bags floating up and down, up and down, aren't they cool? Just let me watch the bags. Let me be. Let me rest. This is a safe place. This is a safe place …

——————

I am awake.

Whuh—shit—where am I? *St. Giles psych ward.* What time is it? *Look at your watch, it's on the table.* Fumbling … here it is. Too dark. Can't see. *Put on your glasses.* Fumble. OK, there. No, still can't see. Maybe I can go back to sleep. I'll try. Close eyes … no … oh no … no, please no, the tide, the sick pitiless buzzing electric tide, it's rising, rising, pouring over the ruined levee of my sleep. What do I do? What do I do? *Get up, find Nurse Wendy.* No, no, I'm too tired. I don't want to know what time it is, maybe it's close to dawn, I'll just lie here, lie stone-still in the nightmare semidarkness and let the tide rip, I can do it, I've done it before, I'm so tired, so tired … please no … *Get up! She's right out there, she said she would be there all night. Ask her for help. GET UP, DAMMIT!* Fine, fine, Christ, stop shouting at me, I'll try! I'll try. Sitting up. Oh, Jesus, it's cold. Oh Jesus, why am I alive? I just want to rest, I thought I could rest here in the hospital, but it's the same, the storm demons are here, they followed me here, I can't escape, I'll never escape, never, never … *Stand up!* OK. Here I go. God, the floor is bouncing hard, up down up down up … *Move. Walk to the door.* Shuffling, trembling, through the pool of tears and out the door, turn, look at the clock on the dayroom wall. One thirty. One thirty a.m. Just as I predicted. It's only one thirty, my god, my god, there is no hope, no hope, my god … *Go find Nurse Wendy. Look, she's right over there, behind the glass. Go tell her you're awake. Ask her to help you. Ask her.*

I stumble to the nurses' window. A fuzzy figure slides it open.

"Hi, Jocelyn! How are you doing?"

"Bad. I'm awake. I feel bad. Really bad."

"Do you want some Ativan?"

"OK. I guess so. Yes."

She says to wait there, she'll get it for me. I am scared at the thought of a benzo, I recall what happened at the healing center with the clonazepam, but at this point it doesn't really matter, does it? *In for a penny, in for a pound. My mother said, take everything that's going.* I clutch the ledge under the window and wait, throat burning limbs shaking eyes blurring ears throbbing floor bouncing brain screaming in exhaustion, misery, fear. The window slides open again, the fuzzy figure says to hold out my wristband for the scanner then hands me a doll-sized paper cup with a pill in it. A cup of water follows. I swallow the pill, say "thanks," and shuffle back to my room. I use the toilet, squinting against the bathroom glare. Then (I guess) I turn off the light and get back into bed, but I don't remember any of that; all I remember is waking up again to the exact same semidarkness, thinking "oh no, oh Jesus please no," fumbling for my glasses, getting up, stumbling out to the dayroom, turning to look at the clock on the wall, and—

(Holy Mother of God) "It's ... it's ten past six!"

I turn to look out the steel-meshed windows. In the distance, above the folded mountaintops, streaks of rose and gold on a pearlescent gray sky are announcing the break of day. I turn again and see Nurse Wendy in her royal-blue scrubs coming toward me, blonde hair shining, kind eyes smiling.

"Yes," she says, "look at that! You slept all the way through!"

I slept all the way through.

I slept all the way through.

I feel like death in a ditch—but I slept all the way through.

CHAPTER 9

A MAD TEA PARTY

The Hollywood movies on which the general public bases its conception of the loony bin—*Cuckoo's Nest, Snake Pit, Girl Interrupted,* and so on—are depictions not of psychiatric wards but of psychiatric hospitals, which are quite different things. Psych wards exist in the upper circles of Dante's Inferno, psych hospitals in the lower. (Rehab centers and halfway houses offer a range of purgatorial experiences.) The main distinction between psych wards and psych hospitals is that the former are waystations while the latter, once called insane asylums, are residences, designed to house folks whose illnesses have been judged both dangerous and intractable. Mental patients given to violence—usually men—are commonly sent straight to a psych hospital; for everyone else, the first stop is a psych ward, a.k.a. behavioral health unit, where the typical stay is three to seven days.* Patients who don't improve within, say, two to three weeks may be transferred to a hospital for longer term, more assiduous care.

Current US law says you can't be held against your will in any sort of mental health facility as long as you've committed no crime and are not a threat to yourself or others; once you're in such a facility, though, what's "against your will" isn't so clear, because "your will" becomes a tenuous, wafting thing, like wisps

---

* Google says fifteen days, but that's because they fail to recognize the ward vs. hospital distinction.

of smoke from a lost camper's frantic attempts to start a fire with two sticks. The strapping on of the blood-pressure cuff, the invitation to join the group, the entrance of the dinner cart at five: are these events against your will, in line with your will, or just bricks in the solid wall of reality before which the fluid will must give way? Does your will have any substance, any direction, any force at all? Do the people in charge perceive your will, and would it matter if they did? You don't know. It's very distressing.

Now let's look at it from the other side. You are a nurse or counselor working in a psych ward. During each twelve-hour shift you must supervise a brood of basket cases who are, for the most part, limply malleable but also given to strange fixations; desperate for help but equally desperate to leave; numbly taciturn but liable to cry or shout at the least provocation. You must not only supervise these non-alert, uncooperative, and poorly groomed individuals but also try to kindle in them a spark of courage and hope. All this in three to seven days, on average, which isn't long enough for the typical psychiatric drug to take effect.

Given such challenges, we might expect Madland to be staffed by medical tyrants with a need for control swollen over time from self-protective severity to monstrous malice. And maybe some psych wards *are* overseen by monsters; mine, however, was not. Were there bossy-pants? Yes, a couple. Sadistic Nurse Ratcheds? No, not one. Because life in the loony bin, it turns out, isn't a horror movie. It's a tea party: the longest, dullest, weirdest tea party ever laid on. The party hosts are gracious, yet strict on etiquette; the party guests are mostly amiable, though eccentric. There are plentiful snacks and beverages, sedate parlor games, and frequent queries as to one's health. Ambitions are tightly circumscribed. Early departures aren't done.

And there's a schedule, steady as a rolling tea trolley but subject to odd lurches and wobbles. Here's how my fourth full day in the ward (or was it the fifth?) played out.

7 a.m. The screechy rumble of the breakfast cart makes for a harsh awakening. Thanks to the clonazepam, I'm now sleeping through the night, sort of. On my second evening Nurse Wendy gave me, along with my other meds, the little blue benzo pill: one full milligram as prescribed by the doctors, none of that zero-point-two-five nonsense. An hour later I turned out the light, got into bed, lay down, and … (Wait. What's different? The bed. It's not moving. The bed's not moving. THE BED'S NOT MOVING!) Into my mind swam an image of Dr. Cook from nearly three years ago, Dr. Cook in his bright red shirt standing in his doggy daycare yoga physical therapy studio, shrugging as he said, "The only thing that works for mal debarquement vertigo is Valium." *Well, hey, Knave of Hearts: you were right.*

But despite the improved sleep, mornings remain very bad indeed. I summon a clench-jawed, blank-eyed faith *Get up!* (I can't, I can't, please) *Don't think, just do it!* in order to heave my body to sitting, then standing, after which I pull on my grippy socks with the smiley faces, shuffle to the bathroom, pee, wash hands, shuffle out to the dayroom with stringless pajama pants loose but not dropping, approach the hulking white metal cart with its meal trays in slots, search blearily for mine, *it's the one with the cup of hot water and the mint teabag no not that one no not that one* (It's not here!!) *don't be silly see there it is,* extract the tray, carry it to a table by the windows, sit, fumble with the plastic-wrapped package of black plastic fork and spoon—no knives of any kind are allowed here—and commence scooping, chewing, swallowing. I am no longer panicky, but I am still scared. And depressed. And sick. God, I'm so sick.

A couple of the other patients are also up and breakfasting. Lindsey the Coloring Girl is at her round table in the back corner, nibbling toast and sipping coffee; Sam the Cast-Footed Guy is hunched over his tray of pancakes and eggs at the long table in front of the bookcase. We eat in separate silence, until … 7:30, end of quiet hours, time for bandana guy, aka the Mad Hatter, his name is Joe, to emerge and cross to the TV. He flops down and clicks the remote. A NASCAR whine drills my skull. Mad Hatter Joe, maybe because he's been here longer than anyone else, is king of the remote. One week hence, I will have seniority and I will be queen of the remote, but I don't know that now; all I know right now is, I could do without Joe.

8 a.m. Nurse Kim, whom I'm just starting to distinguish from Nurse Annette, both with their oatmeal-colored bobs, calls us to morning meeting. Here come Joe, Lindsey, Sam, and Richie the Puzzle Guy, skirting the 1980s dorm furniture, gathering round. Here comes Tessa, the petite woman with cascades of dark curly hair; she's hard of hearing, off and on, whether from physical or emotional causes I don't know; it wouldn't be polite to ask why. And here's Miranda, who arrived the other day: chatty, big boned, probably in her 50s, a devout Christian with thin gray hair scraped back in a ponytail. Miranda naps a lot and lacks teeth.

"I left my teeth at home," she told me and Lindsey yesterday at dinner.

"Don't you need them to eat?" I asked.

"Nah," she said, "I just stick to soft food, it's fine." Her gummy smile is like a gryphon's.

Slowly we assemble in the central square of chairs and couches. Morning meeting here is much shorter than the one at the healing center, the expectations much lower: we need only state our name and one goal for the day. Lindsey says she wants to finish her book, a thriller. "Is it scary?" asks Nurse Kim. Lindsey says yes, it's very scary, she's enjoying it, and Nurse Kim smiles and says, "That's good." Richie, who is being discharged this afternoon (wow, people actually leave here, *no don't think about that now*), says he plans to finish his puzzle. Mad Hatter Joe and Cast-foot Sam both announce their intent to stay positive and trust Jesus. Miranda the Gryphon updates us on her quest to get into a group home here in town; she has been on the phone with her social worker, and they're making progress, she says.

Possibly Deaf Tessa, who is sitting as usual with knees to her chest and the alert-but-vague expression of a forest creature—she won't wear a mask, and the staff don't force her—seems unaware that it's her turn.

"Tessa?" says Nurse Kim. "*Tessa.* TESSA!"

Tessa jumps, dark eyes widening in her gaunt but pretty face. "Huh?"

"*Do you have a goal for the day?*"

"Uh—what?" Her voice is clipped, distracted.

"A GOAL FOR THE DAY!"

"Oh! No, no, I don't really have a goal. No, no. I don't think I have a goal."

"OK, that's fine."

"What?"

"THAT'S FINE. THANK YOU, TESSA."

Now they're all looking at me. I am prepared. Since my first morning, I've remained in pajamas all day, and no one has remarked; nevertheless, I sense that daytime pajama-wearers are considered grubby defeatists, and I'm determined not to be seen as such, so I take a deep breath: "Hi, I'm Jocelyn. My goal for the day is to get dressed."

Nurse Kim gives me a nod and a curt "Fine." (What, isn't that a big enough goal? Christ, what do you people want from me?) Next, we rise for easy stretches, then, "OK," Kim says, "let's make it a great day!" *Let's make it a great day* is the psych ward equivalent of *We're so glad you're here.* A dopey catchphrase, but is there a better one? Aloha … Go team … Anchors aweigh? As the group disperses, I'm feeling miffed at my goal's tepid reception.

8:30 a.m. After morning meeting, it's meal-ordering time. The kitchen likes the mental patients to order lunch, dinner, and next day's breakfast in advance, so you need to have your list of selections ready before you call. When on my first morning Nurse Annette gave me a menu and explained the procedure, I was overwhelmed; now, with four days' experience under my belt, I pull my chair up to my credenza, cross my legs, and study the trifold sheet, impressed anew at its diner-like scope: everything from burgers to salads, fish to fajitas. For each meal we can order one entrée and as many sides, desserts, and drinks as we want. ("So awesome!" says Gryphon Miranda. "I'm getting two desserts!") For hospital food, I have to say, it's all pretty good. I use a stubby pencil—there are no pens, and for some reason no erasers, but blunt pencil stubs are plentiful—to note my choices on the back of a coloring sheet of the Virgin Mary. Then I return to the dayroom to seek out the ward phone: that same object with which Mad Hatter Joe terrorized me during my extreme-pacing session on evening one. Unlike our own phones, which are locked away, the ward phone is freely available in the daytime: the only restrictions are no hogging and no taking it to the bedrooms. Once you're done, etiquette says you offer it to someone else. *In hindsight,* Sane Me muses, *Joe was probably just trying to be polite.*

I punch in 3455 for the kitchen, and a pleasant voice takes my orders. I used to love room service. Too bad I don't love things anymore. When I'm finished, I give the phone to Lindsey.

This is also the hour for morning vitals and meds. By eight-fifty I've managed to get dressed and am huddled on a couch in jeans, maroon sweater, and fleecy black hat, staring at a page of My Book, which still may as well be written in Sanskrit. I hear the glide of the vitals cart and, "Good morning, Jocelyn!" It's Nurse Craig, the day nurse assigned to me today.

I like Nurse Craig. On my very first morning he approached as I sat with head down, rocking, Elephant hugged to my chest. "Hi there!" he said. "Can you rate your anxiety level?"

"Um … maybe … seven?"

"Oh, *that's* not good! Let me get you some Ativan." Off he went and brought me back the pill in its paper cup. This anxiety rating system has merit, I thought as I swallowed. "Hey, what a cool elephant!" he said, and acted interested when I recounted how I made her myself from a kit, 45 years ago in junior high. Later, I asked him for my fleecy hat: "Please, I need it," I said, "to muffle the noise." He found it among my stored things and handed it over.

Now he rolls the cart into position beside me. "OK if I take your vitals?" I nod, doff the hat, and stick out an arm for the cuff, finger for the clip, forehead for the thermometer. Most of the nurses make you come to the desk and don't ask permission to poke and prod; only a few, like Craig, will roll the cart to you and ask. Their polite requests are analogous to the towel screens: ceremonial, because the procedures involved are non-optional, but appreciated nonetheless.

9:30 a.m. Snacks! In comes the snack cart with the pudding and juice cups, chips and fruit. I never look up in time to see it emerge. Whence does it come? Who stocks it? There are spaces outside the ward that may as well be other universes: inaccessible, unseen, unfathomable.

I know what's in the conference room to the left of the main entrance; I've been there for semiweekly "team meetings" during which I sit at the head of a long table, facing the water-ice machine on the counter at the other end, trying not to cry while a doctor, a couple of nurses, and a counselor interrogate and observe me. (Although I occupy the head seat, nobody mistakes me for the team leader.) When not in use, the conference room is locked, but it's the place where, in the evening, we patients may be permitted to go and use our own phones for ten minutes. Across from it is the locked door to the tiny staffroom through which I entered on my first evening. Off in a corner there's a sunroom with straw mats and a cagelike steel-mesh wall, thicker than the window mesh, that admits fresh air; this room, too, is normally locked, except when weather permits it to be open for a few hours at midday. Down the back corridor is the door to the laundry room, plus a few mystery doors, all locked. Up front are the fearsome double doors of the main entrance, which one never approaches because *ALARM WILL SOUND.*

And there is one more locked door, right of the nurses' station, to a room that (I think) is meant to confine badly behaved patients. Behind that door, I feel sure, is my new worst nightmare: Padded cell? Lobotomy chamber? Room 101, the Rats' Revenge?

Maybe it's where they store the snack cart.

10:00 a.m. After Snack comes Group: mandatory, twice a day. Claims of being sick and unable to attend are regarded with skepticism. Yesterday after morning meds I went to my room, feeling awful, thinking I would just lie down for a moment and rest my eyes ... only to be jolted awake by a smack on the ass and, "Get up! Time for Group!" The smacker was Nurse Debra, the boss nurse. Debra's a martinet, but she's not so bad really; she reminds me of my old ballet teachers, with their propensity to beat time, and occasionally one's limbs, with slim wooden canes. In my head, Nurse Debra is the Duchess.

But Debra the Duchess doesn't lead Group; that's the job of Counselors Paula and Nadine. Nadine is the Red Queen, with a smooth auburn bob and a brisk manner; she wears leather boots and tight dark-wash jeans. Paula, who is on today, is the White Queen, with fluffy white shoulder-length hair and an air of gentle grievance; she wears sneakers and woolen shawls. I prefer Paula to Nadine because, despite her injured aura, Paula gives the impression of enjoying her job, while Nadine always seems to be hoping something better will come along.

"OK, folks, Group!" says Paula with a light clap of the hands. "Let's turn off the TV."

Mad Hatter Joe clicks the remote (blessed quiet!) and the seven of us move to the long table in front of the bookcase, pull out chairs, take our seats. So far, and happily, Group has demanded no bag puppets, no origami, no "projects"; instead we hunch over worksheets, writing thoughts about coping skills or letters to ourselves from our Higher Power, then reading our responses aloud—if we want to, that is, for although our presence is required, sharing is not. The women participate more than the men, and some of the stories are wrenching. Yesterday, for example, Lindsey told us about how when she was a little girl her brothers would make her run to and fro in the yard while they shot at her with a BB gun. The correct response to such shares isn't finger snaps, thank goodness, but silence or an affirmative murmur. (At my very first Group, I wrote and shared rambling thoughts about the terrors of chronic vertigo, which Mad Hatter Joe judged "profound," causing my opinion of him to tick upward.) Next the counselor might offer a psychological insight or two, then someone else might share a story; no one, however, engages in games of top-my-trauma. At the Mad Tea Party, it's understood we're all equal: in sickness, in suffering, in numb quotidian strength.

11:30 a.m. The fearsome double doors swing open with a mechanical clunk-whoosh and the meals tower re-enters, screaming *institutional setting* as the orderly trundles it across the linoleum. There is some, not pleasure, let's just say satisfaction, in seeing it arrive and knowing Group will now end and we will have the lunch we ordered, the lunch we chose. I retrieve my tray of chef's salad, milk, and mint teabag, Lindsey her sandwich, chips, and coffee, and Miranda her soup and two desserts. The three of us sit together, eating our meal with our plastic forks and spoons and our teeth or gums as applicable. Things are not desperately bad.

1 p.m. Patient discharges generally happen after lunch. Richie is the one leaving today; he has finished his jigsaw puzzle, for which he received congratulations from White Queen Paula during Group. Now he heads out, accompanied by Nurse Craig, who carries his stuff in a big translucent pink garbage bag. As he exits, he offers an indiscriminate wave to us, the Left Behind. We all wave back, except Miranda the Gryphon, who is napping in her room.

Napping is a popular post-lunch activity. On my first afternoon, I was sitting at the back table with Lindsey, both of us coloring, Elephant quietly observing, when all at once I woke up—and realized I'd been asleep, yes, had actually nodded off right there at the table. Glancing at the wall clock, I realized I'd been out for almost ten minutes. *Ativan, Ativan, Ativan be praised!* That evening, during own-phone time, I sent an email to friends and family with this report:

> BIG NEWS ... i had a nap today!!!! Dozed off for 10 mins withought terror. I was pretty shocked. First time in 3 mnoths. I can't describe the joy this brought me. Just to nap. Amazing.*

Since then, I've been on clonazepam. "Ativan is your fast-acting med, for acute anxiety," Nurse Craig explained, "and the clonazepam is your smooth, long-lasting med, which you'll take morning and evening"—with the result that I now never *fail* to fall asleep, several times a day, doesn't matter where I am or what's going on. I've taken to carrying a pillow to my seats around the dayroom, ready for the inevitable conk-out.

---

* Years on, a friend said it was this email that made her grasp the direness of my situation. "There were typos," she said, "and all-caps, and *four* exclamation points. It was so unlike you!"

"… Jocelyn. Jocelyn." Someone is shaking my shoulder quite roughly. "Jocelyn! Wake up." I open my eyes to a man's face looming across my field of vision. (Unh … where am I? What is) *St. Giles psych ward.* (Oh right but who is that man and why is his face sideways) *You're lying on the couch in front of the TV. You fell asleep. That's Dr. Taylor.*

"Jocelyn? Can you wake up?" His voice sounds tense.

"Huh? Oh. Sorry. Yeah." I don't want to wake up. The pillow is so nice and soft.

"It's time for our visit. Are you feeling OK?"

"Yeah. Uh … I'm awake. I can … yes." I raise myself to sitting. Dr. Taylor is kneeling on the floor, peering at me, his brow furrowed. He takes my wrist and checks my pulse. "You OK?" he repeats, and hands me my water cup. I take a sip. Then he helps me to my feet, and I follow him to the conference room, pulling up my mask, Elephant tucked in the crook of my arm. Why all the fuss? I wonder. Dude, I was just napping.

On returning to the dayroom, I rejoin Lindsey at the coloring table. She says, "Did you know the doctor was trying to wake you up? You wouldn't wake up."

"Really?"

"Yeah, he was, like, shaking you and calling your name for a long time, but you wouldn't wake up. I was sort of freaked out."

"Huh. Did you think I was dead?"

"Ha-ha, yeah, maybe!"

"Nah. Not dead."

We both smile through our masks and resume coloring. I do *feel* dead—well, half-dead—but since half-dead in hospital is better than a hundred percent alive in hell, I won't complain, and neither, in my opinion, should the doctors. "Soft food is fine," said Miranda the Gryphon. As far as I'm concerned, soft pillows and hard, hard naps are fine, too.

2 p.m. For afternoon Group, White Queen Paula has brought her manila envelope of pictures, dozens of them: people, animals, plants, landscapes, street scenes, all cut from magazines, all a bit grimy and tattered. Gathered at the long table are Lindsey, Miranda, Tessa, and me. Sam and Joe haven't joined us; Sam is having his cast changed, who knows what Joe's excuse is.

Paula likes this activity. With happy energy, she spreads the worn clippings on the table and tells us to peruse them and take one, one that speaks to us. Then we write down our thoughts about our selection. Then we go around the circle and share.

Lindsey has chosen a picture of a sunrise. "I guess I'm being discharged on Wednesday," she says. "I sort of feel like the sun is rising; like it's a new day."

Paula adjusts her shawl and smiles. "Great, Lindsey. How are you feeling about that?"

"Good. I'm a little nervous about going home, though."

"And it's perfectly normal to be a little nervous," Paula says. "Perfectly normal."

Miranda has picked a picture of a dog. "I picked this one because it reminds me of *my* dog, Celeste," she says. "I had to give her to the shelter before I came here. She's such a sweetie. I miss her so much. I'm gonna get her back, though, it's just temporary at the shelter. If I can get into Casa Rosa, they'll let me have her there. I didn't want to give her up, but I had no choice, I mean, after the demon came into my house and came into my body, *here*" (she points to a spot on her abdomen, her tone upbeat, informative) "… I knew there was no way I could stay in that house by myself. Wow, it was scary. Celeste barked and growled, she knew there was something wrong. Demons, man, they are no joke! I tried to make it go away, I prayed to Jesus to help me, and he did, he helped me, but I can't go back to that house, it wouldn't be safe for me. I'm getting new meds for my bipolarism, I think they're working. I hope my social worker can get me into Casa Rosa. It's the perfect situation, cuz they'll let me keep Celeste. I miss her so much." She looks down at the dog picture, her expression soft. "She's such a sweetie."

"I really hope it works out for you," Paula says. "Thank you for sharing that, Miranda." She turns to Tessa, who is gazing into space, hands in her lap, a photo of a scarlet hibiscus on the table before her. "Tessa, will you tell us about the picture you chose?"

"What?"

"*Will you tell us about the picture you chose?*"

Tessa leans forward, pushing long dark curls behind her left ear. "Huh?"

"TELL US WHY YOU CHOSE THE FLOWER."

"Oh! Sure. I chose this flower because, um, I think, I don't know … yeah …" There is a lengthy pause in which we all sit frozen in suspense. "… I just liked it."

"Do you want to share what you like about it?"

"What?"

"WHAT DO YOU LIKE ABOUT IT?"

"I dunno. It's just, like … pretty. Also, can I say something?"

"Yes, of course."

"Huh? Oh, OK. Yesterday somebody stole my lunch. I didn't get any lunch. Somebody took it. But I'm gonna ask to see the security cameras, because the person will be on there, and then I'll see, I'll know who took my lunch." Her eyes, gazing into space, burn with wrathful hurt. "And then I'll report them, and they'll be in trouble. They probably think they can get away with it, but they can't, because I know there are security cameras, and—"

Paula breaks in: "OK, Tessa, let's address that later. Thank you for sharing."

"What?"

"THANK YOU FOR SHARING!"

"Oh! Sure, no problem." Tessa sits back, the lunch thief seemingly forgotten.

Now it's my turn to talk about my chosen picture of a giraffe. As usual, I've penciled out my thoughts at length and am ready to deliver. I begin to read aloud:

> Giraffes are not considered one of the "Big Five" safari animals—the Big Five are Elephant, Lion, Leopard, Water Buffalo, and Rhinoceros. But Giraffes were my mother's favorite animal, and she transmitted that love to me. When you see a giraffe in a zoo, you get no sense of how beautiful they are when they run.

Suddenly I'm crying, I don't know why, maybe it was Miranda's dog, or my mother, or maybe just, you know, giraffes. (God, will I ever function normally again? *Don't think about that.*) Paula shoves the tissue box at me. I pull one and continue, weeping:

> My mother was always sad when she saw giraffes in a zoo, because they need to run. [*sniff*] I feel a bit like a giraffe in a zoo, because I used to be able to run and now it's like I'm [*cough*] in a cage. But maybe my spirit can still be a running giraffe [*snuffle*], running over the Serengeti, in a state of freedom. I'm not sure how to achieve that.

I blow my nose and say, "That's it."

"Thank you for sharing, Jocelyn," says Paula. "That was very beautiful."

"Sure, no problem."

3 p.m. Behind me I hear the rumble of the snack cart, signaling the end of Group. "Snacks are here!" says Paula. The relief is palpable as we rise and hurry to claim our munchies. I'm still eschewing junk food, but Sane Me has decided to reclassify pudding as not-junk-food (*It's milk, right?*) so I select a container and carry it to the TV zone, where I take a seat behind Joe and Tessa, peel off the foil top, and spoon up the vanilla-yellow goo as CNN pundits analyze the election. Biden, they're saying, has won Pennsylvania. Miranda comes and sits down beside me: "They're saying there was fraud." She peels off the top of her Jell-o cup and digs in. "I dunno. I think there was, probably. But we gotta accept it, right? We gotta accept it and move on."

"Yes," I say. "We've got to accept it and move on."

4 p.m. Recreation, like Group, is mandatory, though not *as* mandatory: the TV must be off, but if you're napping in your room, they won't come in and slap you awake. In theory there are a number of possible activities, including board games, cards, nerf balls, and jigsaw puzzles; in practice, since none of us (except Richie the Puzzle Guy, now departed) is up to such efforts, there is "art." The counselor on duty unlocks the big cabinet under the counter and from it pulls yet another cart, this one crammed full of trays, jars, and bundles: watercolor paints, paint brushes, water cups, pastels, more crayons, colored pencils, rolls of paper, and even scissors—a lawful chaos of tired but potentially dangerous art supplies. Sitting at the long table, under the cautious eye of Paula the White Queen or Nadine the Red, we paint or draw. Rustles of paper underscore quiet utterances: "Are you done with that brown pencil?" "Could I have the pastels, please?" The atmosphere is different from the healing center's craft room: less holiday camp, more monastery scriptorium. The only one of us who shows any artistic ability is Tessa.

Outside the steel-meshed windows, the afternoon light fades.

5 p.m. Clunk-whoosh go the main doors. Rumble-screech goes the meals tower. We help Paula put away the art supplies and go to fetch our dinners. This time, everyone eats together at the long table. The conversation is patchy, focused on the food. Joe and Tessa finish quickly, bus their trays, and repair to opposite ends of the TV couch to watch Duck Dynasty.

Half an hour later, Elephant and I are back at the coloring table. I'm using an annoyingly dry green marker to fill in the hem of an angel's robe when Tessa approaches and seats herself in the chair next to me. In her hand is a white paper cup with a lid, one of the small-tall ones that come with our mealtime coffees and teas.

"Hi," she says, leaning in quite close.

"Hi." I feel crowded, nervous.

"I made this for you." She hands me the cup, and I see it has a piece of white paper wrapped around it, awkwardly folded and Scotch-taped, with designs drawn in colored pencil: a magenta-and-black scalloped border, a multicolored bursting blossom reminiscent of a peony, a couple of birdwing silhouettes, and a black outline of a puffy cloud with two fat raindrops falling from its edge. It's the picture she was drawing during recreation.

"You know how you were crying before? In Group? You had, like, tears, tears on your face?" She touches her cheek with her fingertips.

I nod. "Yes, I was."

"I was wondering ..." She looks off into space, back again. "... why were you sad?"

"I don't know."

"What?"

"I DON'T KNOW."

"Oh. See, I made this for you, so maybe you won't cry anymore." She points to the cup. "See, the cloud is raining, this is rain, the rain is watering the flower, see the sky, the sky is up here, sometimes we get sad, and the sun is behind the cloud ..." She continues for some time, pointing out the elements of her design, an earnest rambling discourse on rain and sun and tears, and although I don't understand more than a quarter of what she says, I have no difficulty grasping the basic message: *I made this for you, so maybe you won't cry anymore.*

6:30 p.m. The night is in, the ceiling lights fluorescing as we gather for evening meeting, during which we restate our morning goal and say whether we achieved it. Nurse Annette is the meeting leader this time; after I say my goal was to get dressed and that I did in fact get dressed, her eyes crinkle with approval as she says, "Oh, right, you've been staying in your loungewear, haven't you? But today you put on street clothes. That's great!"

See? says Sane Me. *Told you it was a good goal.*

7:00 p.m. Laden with coats and handbags, trailing whiffs of cold November air, a pair of night nurses enter through the fearsome double doors and stride past the TV, heading for the back corridor where (I guess) there must be a changing room. From Joe, Sam, Lindsey, and Miranda comes a chorus of "Hi, ladies!" and a flurry of waves. The nurses wave back, cheerful. I make a mental note that greeting the night nurses when they arrive is the polite thing to do; of course it is, why haven't I done it so far? But this is the first night I've noticed them arrive. Did they sneak in through another door on previous nights? Or did I simply not register their arrival?

Tonight, I remember with sorrow, there is no Nurse Wendy; she works the night shift Wednesday to Saturday, and this is Sunday. On duty tonight are Nurses Colleen and Yvonne. Nurse Colleen is youngish, with pale skin and dark eyebrows. Nurse Yvonne is a tall stout Black woman with gold-wire-rimmed glasses and hair flecked with gray. Having changed into their scrubs—light blue for Colleen, royal for Yvonne—the two of them come from the back room and join the day nurses in the enclosure. None of us waves this time; they have morphed from *ladies* whom we greet as equals to *nurses* whose status relative to us isn't quite clear, but who we know are very busy and must get on with their work, which during shift change means sitting in their fishbowl with their tablets and clipboards discussing— what? Us, presumably.

New patients are often brought in at this evening hour, a practice that in my case I chalked up to bad timing but that I now see is likely standard, for during shift change there are a full five nurses (three day and two night) available to deal with a distraught, possibly agitated newbie. "This is the worst part," said Nurse Annette on my first evening as I sat sobbing in the wheelchair, and she was right, intake is horrible. I think it must be stressful for the nurses, too. If the patient is male, does the security guard stay for the strip search? Probably.

Nurse Colleen comes over to say there's a new patient with "medical challenges" who needs a room with a full-on hospital bed, which means a reorg for us old-timers. The first room in the row of four, currently Tessa's, is the one with the hospital bed, so the newcomer must go there. Tessa must move into my room, and I will overleap the third room, which is Miranda and Lindsey's, and take the fourth room, lately vacated by Richie. (Joe and Sam in the fifth room, by the bookcase, are unaffected.) I know from reports that the other bedrooms are if anything too warm, whereas mine has remained freezing no matter how they fiddle with the thermostat. Warmth will be nice. I feel a little bad for Tessa, though. Why aren't they simply moving her to Room 4? *Because they need Tessa to stay in the panopticon,* Sane Me explains, *and they think you can be trusted farther away. It's a compliment, really.* Moving my stuff to Room 4 doesn't take long, and as I tote the clothes and toiletries I don't bother to conceal my secret hoard of juice cups, now with apple as well as cranberry.

The newbie, who looks to be elderly or maybe just very sick, arrives in a wheelchair around 7:30 and is trundled straight into Room 1. Later we learn that her name is Bonnie. As I sit with the others watching TV, I can see through the half-open door the nurses bustling about, maneuvering equipment, getting Bonnie into bed, and into my mind comes the voice of Dr. Greene: *You know, I have vertigo patients in wheelchairs who can't even walk, your case sounds pretty mild.* I suppose after all he was right, and I am grateful I can walk and am not in a wheelchair and I get to be at the end of the row with a modicum of privacy, and yet, and yet … after they turn out Bonnie's light, and gentle snores indicate she has fallen asleep, sound asleep at 7:55 pm, I feel a twinge of envy.

8 p.m. Snack cart! Right on time. I pick out a granola bar and take it to the coloring table, where I finish the angel's robe, careful not to drop too many crumbs as I eat.

Then it's time for vitals check. Nurse Yvonne calls me to the desk; I'm in her charge tonight. As she reads out my numbers (temp normal, pulse ox normal, blood pressure down in the zombie zone as usual), I hear what seems to me a Caribbean accent, bringing to mind a childhood era when I lived with my diplomat parents in Kingston, Jamaica. The voice is warmly familiar: the sound of a Neverland of bicycles, palm trees, and orange Fanta. I consider remarking on it, decide not to, then return to the coloring table and select another picture of an indeterminate biblical figure.

10 p.m. Nurse Colleen signals bedtime by clicking off the television, but evening is still my best time and I'm loath to turn in before I must. I take a shower in my new bathroom, noting with approval that the water pressure is just as strong as in the old bathroom, then remove my contacts—yesterday they let me have my folding hairbrush with tiny built-in plastic mirror, making it unnecessary to peer at my eyeballs in the darkened window—put on my pajamas, and wander out to the dayroom, thinking I might color again for a bit. Nurse Colleen is in the fishbowl. Nurse Yvonne is sitting at the outer desk, doing paperwork. Seized by a sense of wild daring, I approach her.

"Hi … hi, sorry, can I ask you something?"

"Yes?"

"I was just wondering, um … are you Jamaican?"

She shakes her head. "No. I'm Nigerian. I was born in Nigeria."

I take a step back. Sane Me, suddenly, is up in my face shouting *What the hell?! Could you be any ruder? God, why don't you just take a marker and write DUMB RACIST across your forehead* (I'm sorry I'm sorry I didn't mean to be rude I'll fix it I'm sorry I'll explain) *Yeah you'd better explain! Good lord, didn't your mother teach you better than that* (Yes she did I'm sorry I'm sorry I'll fix it I'll fix it right away)

"Oh! Wow, Nigeria." I can feel my face burning. "I just thought, because the thing is, I grew up in Jamaica, well I mean I lived there for a few years, and I thought maybe your accent was Jamaican, that's the only reason I asked, but, um … Nigeria. Wow. That's cool."

Jesus, stop talking. Just stop!

Yvonne is smiling at me through her mask, and her eyes behind the gold-rimmed glasses are benevolent. "Yes, I came here as a little girl. My mother's family are all still there, in Nigeria."

"Oh, I see, that's nice. Well, thanks." I turn around and hurry back to my room, climb onto the bed, yank the covers over my legs.

What a gaffe! What a disaster! Now she hates me because I'm a rich white bitch. "Hey there, brown-skinned lady, are you Jamaican?" Ohmigod, cringe. I'm the worst.

Still … I'm crazy. *That you are.* Don't I get a pass because I'm crazy? I think I should, a small pass at least. *Fine, here's your pass.* But is she angry? *Don't be ridiculous.* She didn't seem angry. In fact, she didn't even seem miffed. And why would she be?

Why would she care what a crazy person says to her? Anyway, I was only trying to connect; "only connect," that's what they say in that book, I forget which one, "only connect." *It's not your job to connect, sweetie.* Right, right, my job is to try and get well, and her job is to help me get well. *Think, now. Think.* OK, I'm thinking … Yvonne is a nurse. She sees me as a patient, *her* patient. When mental patients try to connect, even clumsily, that's a sign they're getting better, right? Five days ago I was barely able to speak, let alone initiate a conversation, and now look at me, I can walk straight up to an authority figure and say something extremely stupid. That's progress, right? Yes. I think that is progress.

Now you're starting to get it says Sane Me as I scrunch down under the covers, breathing in the warm antiseptic air of the new room that looks exactly like the old room, bed legs bolted to the floor and everything. *Yes,* she says, *I really think you're starting to get it.* I've added another book, a historical mystery novel set in Egypt with a picture of pyramids and palm trees on its cover, to the meticulously arranged collection of items on the bedside table. I reach for this, My Other Book, and open it to page two.

CHAPTER 10

QUEEN OF THE REMOTE

~~~~~~~~~~~

Y ou've got depression," said Dr. Taylor. "You're crying."
        I stared at his stethoscope, needing a moment to pro-
cess his meaning—not "crying right now," but "crying on a regular basis," what was that, the present habitual tense?—and to
reflect with annoyance that the nurses must have reported my
afternoon lie-on-bed-and-sob sessions, which, seeing as they
were prompted by exhausted sadness rather than crazed anxiety,
I had been indulging in with some relief. The day was Thursday,
November twelfth, my eighth day in the ward, and Dr. Taylor
had joined me on a dayroom couch for a consultation.

"Crying," he repeated, his mien solemn.

I toyed with the idea of telling him I didn't mind crying,
that crying was better than suicide planning, and moreover that
scientific research indicates tears are good for purging stress
chemicals, but it was all too much.

"I know," I said.

"The anxiety was masking the depression," he said. "The anxiety isn't your real problem."

"I see." I didn't see, and quite frankly didn't agree, but ...
whatever.

"We need to get the sertraline, that's the Zoloft, up higher.
You're at 75 milligrams now, and we're aiming for at least 100
milligrams. But we have to go slow; it'll take some more time to
get there. So what I'm saying is: Don't leave."

I shook my head. *He thinks you're an eloper, ha-ha! ALARM WILL SOUND.* "No, no, don't worry, I won't leave."

"And when you reach the effective dose, you'll know. OK?" The doctor leaned closer, his expression earnest, and said it again: "You will *know*"—as if to make crystal clear that this knowledge, soon to arrive and impossible to mistake, would be the saving of me.

Turns out, he was right.

I didn't buy that the anxiety was "just masking the depression"—after all, I had Dr. Funar's diagnosis of depression *and* generalized anxiety disorder *and* panic disorder—but when Dr. Taylor said, "You will *know*," it was as if finally, finally, after months of fruitless searching, I'd been given the right eat-me-drink-me, the right bit of mushroom to clutch in my fist and nibble as I proceeded through Madland, secure in the belief that although it might take some time, maybe even a lot of time, the remedy would eventually prove effective and serve as my ticket out of this hellish country I'd been trapped in for, how long? It felt like forever.

You will know. Dr. Taylor stood up, adjusted his stethoscope, told me to make it a great day, and took his leave, heading off to wherever the doctors went when they weren't having very short conversations with us patients.

You will know. Was it a psychiatrist's trick for reaching the subconscious of a control freak like me? Maybe, but if it was a trick, it was a very good trick.

When it happens, you will know. I put aside My Other Book, got off the couch, and went to join morning Group with White Queen Paula and the gang.

————

Lindsey the Coloring Girl had been discharged the day before. In the morning she gave me a makeshift folded paper packet: "Wait to read it till after I've gone," she said. Once the main double doors had clunked shut behind her and her nurse escort,

I retrieved the packet from my room and took it to the coloring table. On the cover was a mandala design in lavender, blue, and gold; below the mandala were four blue flowers, above it the words "Open to read your letter" punctuated by a smiley face. I unfolded the paper to find a long, heartfelt message, which at the time I resolved to treasure but have since somehow lost. I recall, though, that she wrote, "I hope you can smile again soon. I bet you have a beautiful smile." And she concluded with a line from Winnie the Pooh: *You are braver than you believe, stronger than you seem, and smarter than you think.*

Cast-foot Sam and Mad Hatter Joe were both discharged on Thursday. The four of us left behind were Tessa the Possibly Deaf, Miranda the Gryphon, Bonnie of the Wheelchair, and me: Woman with the Stuffed Elephant, as I may have been known.

What with all the departures, I had moved up the ranks and been crowned, by unspoken consensus, Queen of the Remote. Tessa had been around longer, but she never attempted to operate the TV (perhaps because she couldn't hear it), and Miranda and Bonnie, being newer than I, deferred to my selections. Strange, I thought, how the laws of seniority apply even here, though perhaps not so surprising if one looked at it as another example of Mad Tea Party etiquette. Of course, with noble status comes noblesse oblige; if someone joined me on the couch before the flatscreen, I'd ask them politely if they wanted to watch something else.

"No, no," they'd always say, "this is fine."

"Are you sure?" I'd say, making not the slightest move to hand them the clicker. "Would you like the volume louder?"

"No, no, it's totally fine."

"OK, well, just let me know if you want me to change it."

One morning I was sitting alone, brain still heavily fogged with illness and drugs but feeling vaguely proud at being able to follow, more or less, the CNN talking heads as they dissected the BREAKING NEWS that TRUMP SAYS VOTING MACHINES RIGGED, when Counselor Nadine (the Red Queen to Paula's White) arrived for her shift. She walked past me, bootheels clacking, smooth auburn bob gleaming—stopped, frowned at the TV, then turned to frown at me while making button-pressing gestures with her red-nailed thumb.

"Let's turn this off," she snapped. "Find something else. A movie or something."

A flash of fury lit up the brain fog and shot out my eyes like a phaser beam. Nadine stood her ground, unphased. The confrontation lasted only a second, for I knew full well that she was a much more powerful queen than I, and that my arsenal for queen-on-queen battles was limited at best. Slowly, with appropriate dignity, I raised the remote and clicked once—twice—landed on Storage Wars, then lowered my arm, stared straight ahead, and silently dared her to make me change the channel again. Nadine glanced at the screen, still frowning, and walked off.

During morning snack, I described the skirmish to Miranda.

"Nadine can't do that!" she said, her rheumy eyes alight with righteous anger. "She can't tell you not to watch the news, you can watch the news if you want to!"

"I know, right?! Who does she think she is?"

"That's *bull*shit!"

"Right?! Why shouldn't I watch the news? It's my choice!"

"It's *totally* your choice. She can*not* do that."

Obviously Nadine could do that, and more. Nevertheless, it felt good to have a loyal supporter of my regime.

———

Our reduced cohort was soon supplemented by new arrivals. In the wee hours of Friday, I awoke to a person howling in rage or fright, I couldn't tell which. The howls went on for five or ten minutes, then stopped. I was perturbed and lay alert for a long while, but eventually fell back into uneasy dreams. Next morning, when Nurse Colleen came in to roust me out of bed—I was becoming inclined to sleep through breakfast—I asked her what had happened.

"Oh, we had a new patient arrive in the night," she said, shrugging. "Sometimes they're a little agitated. Just the way it goes."

The Howler, it transpired, was a young woman maybe 19 or 20 years of age: frame gangly, skin sallow-tan, brow knit with anxiety. She emerged from the bookcase-adjacent room around nine a.m., dressed in maroon scrubs of a disposable nylon material (the standard issue to inmates who arrived without pajamas), and began pacing fast around the dayroom, back and forth and all around, just as I had on my first evening. Unlike me, though, she was bent on testing every possible point of egress: Down the line of big windows she went, tugging on every handle. Over to the sunroom, which hadn't yet been opened for the day, to jiggle the doorknob. Into her bedroom, whence came a sharp rattle of breakproof glass. Back out to stride around the dayroom and down the laundry-room corridor, checking each locked portal. Her search was obsessive but not psychotic: she steered clear of the alarmed double doors. All the while, the nurses in the fishbowl got on with their work and we patients averted our eyes, courteously.

I'd wanted to comfort Kathy the Mock Turtle during her panic attack. With the Howler, I had no such urge. I knew exactly how she felt, and I empathized, even admired her test-the-exits strategy, which I saw as nuttier but also bolder than my first night's doorstop-rigging maneuvers. Her efforts to cope with incarceration had a swashbuckling ferocity, whereas mine, I thought now, had been pathetically cautious. She was in the ward for just a day or two, during which time she never spoke to anybody, silently signaling that this tea party was not for her. I suppose they had her on a 24-hour hold. I don't recall exactly when or how she left, but I was glad, for her sake, that they didn't make her stay.

————

Vaseline Man, who arrived early Friday evening, was a very different case. A shortish, thirty-something guy with slick dark hair, smooth complexion, and a jovial manner, he walked straight over and introduced himself—"Hello, ladies, I'm Albert!"—to me and Miranda as we sat at the coloring table. I had advanced from indeterminate biblical figures to an intricate abstract design of flowers and leaves, which was taking some time to complete, while Miranda was working on a basic angel. We both said hello to the newbie. He stood for a minute with hands behind his back, watching us, then said: "Lemme ask you a question! Are you saved by Jesus?"

"Yes," said Miranda, looking up and nodding.

"Um," said I, doing neither.

"That's great!" Albert beamed through his facemask. "Can I give you my testimony?"

"No thanks," said Miranda.

"No thanks," said I.

"Oh, OK." Looking a bit crestfallen, he continued to stand there watching us work until Nurse Kim (who was still on day duty, it being only seven p.m.) came and ushered him over to the TV couch. He went without complaint.

Nurse Kim returned and said, "Albert is very religious. He wanted to know if he could share his thoughts with you. I told him you prefer he not do that."

"Thanks." Miranda laughed nervously. "Yeah, I really don't want him talking to me. That stuff creeps me out."

"Same," I said, thinking about yesterday afternoon, when Miranda had sat down beside me and asked if she could give me *her* testimony. When I told her to go ahead, she launched again into the story about the demon invading her home and entering her body, and her dog Celeste barking, and how it had been so awful until she'd prayed to Jesus to banish the demon, which had worked, and the demon had gone, except the demon might still be there, and she might have to find an exorcist, but this sort of case demanded a special type of exorcist that isn't available in New Mexico (*makes sense,* said Sane Me, *it's hard to find good specialists in New Mexico*) —anyway, Miranda said, if I prayed to Jesus he would surely heal me. I said I certainly believed in God (little iffy on Jesus) but felt that, at least in my case, He worked in more prosaic, long-term ways: "Like, He gave me the strength and resources to get into the hospital," I said, "during Covid. And they took my insurance, so, yeah." Miranda said yes, that was true, but she knew the power of Jesus and he was the only one who could heal me. "Thank you, I'll think about it," I said. Seemingly satisfied, she had gone off to take a nap.

I looked over at Albert and Tessa now sitting calmly on opposite ends of the TV couch. Funny, I thought, that Miranda doesn't want to hear the Jesus stuff from Albert. Maybe she sees herself as the expert on the topic, needing no advice. Or maybe she thinks Albert's a fraud.

"He understands," Nurse Kim was saying. "He means well. I don't think he'll bother you. But if he does, just let us know, OK?"

"We will," said Miranda, looking askance at the two on the couch.

The next morning, Albert needed no coaxing to join Group. He seated himself at the long table with a friendly "Morning, folks!" and leaned back at ease, knees splayed. White Queen Paula had gone off to fetch some supplies, so there was a lag before the session could start. Seemingly eager to fill the conversational void, Albert began to chat.

"So how is everybody today?"

Murmurs of *good, good, how're you* from the rest of us at the table.

"I'm good! So we do the group therapy thing, huh? That's cool. I've done it before … it's helpful, right? Talking about our feelings." He turned to Tessa. "You doin' OK, dear?"

"What?" Her forest-creature eyes widened at him.

"Yeah, you're OK. Jesus has got you, right?"

"Huh?"

Reyes, a solid, forthright young woman with armfuls of tattoos who had arrived yesterday, diagnosis unclear, took a swig from her water mug and said, "She can't hear you, dude."

"Oh, right," said Albert, unperturbed. "That's cool, that's cool! I just love to talk about Jesus, you know? He's my lord and savior! Jesus saves!"

Miranda, who seemed in better spirits today, smiled and said, "Praise Jesus."

"You know it! He's everywhere. Even here. Things are pretty good here, right? They have everything. Good food, good medicine, good company, ha-ha!" He sent a grin around the table, then winced and shook his head as if pierced by a sudden painful memory. "They don't have Vaseline, though. Last night I was trying to get them to gimme some Vaseline, and they said I could only have this little teeny jar." He held up his thumb and forefinger an inch apart. "No good! I need a lot of Vaseline. A *lot*."

Curiosity overcame me. "Why do you need so much Vaseline?"

"Vaseline, man! It's the *best*." His face lit up again. "You rub it over your whole body, and it makes your skin super soft. Then when the Rapture comes, or whatever, it lets you slide right up to heaven. It greases you up! Makes you smooth and silky for the judgment day!"

I inspected him for signs of irony and saw none.

"I'm tellin' ya: nothing like Vaseline! I put it *all* over my body. Y'all gotta try it. Seriously, I'm waiting for the Rapture, man! I'm gonna be ready, praise Jesus!"

"Praise him!" said Miranda, flashing a toothless grin over her drooping facemask.

Counselor Paula came bustling back, woolen shawl askew, toting a stack of workbooks. "Sorry for the delay! How is everybody this morning?"

"Great!" said Albert. "We were just talking about Vaseline!"

"Oh?" Paula cast him a doubtful look. "Well ... let's talk about coping skills, shall we? Got some new workbooks for you!" She handed them out, and Group commenced.

Later, Albert and Tessa were again ensconced on the TV couch as Miranda, Reyes, and I finished our lunch at the long table. Albert made a comment; Tessa got on her hands and knees and crawled close to him, as if to hear him better. She stayed in that all-fours position, long dark curls framing her laughing, pretty face, as Albert chatted on, animatedly.

"Jeez, look at that," muttered Miranda through a mouthful of cheese enchiladas.

"What," said Reyes.

Miranda gestured with her chin. "Look at that girl, sticking her butt in the air."

"I thought she was deaf," Reyes said, turning to stare.

"Huh! *She* knows what she's doing. She comes on to all the guys. Sticking her butt in the air. She did it with Joe, now with this dude. And he's eating it up. She better be careful."

Confused, I eyed the two on the couch. Was Tessa really coming on to Albert? Was Albert really eating it up? I'd been assuming they were, like all Madlanders, asexual beings; in light of Miranda's remarks, I suddenly saw two attractive individuals in their mid-thirties who—were this a bar instead of a psych ward—might easily have been on track for a hookup. I recalled that when Tessa took a shower, she'd have a nurse stand outside the curtain and pass her a razor so she could shave her legs. *If you want my body, and you think I'm sexy ...* Rod Stewart warbled in my head. Miranda continued to look daggers, and I wondered again whether her cynicism was born of bitter experience with charming, crazy men: sellers of snake oil, or maybe Vaseline.

————

Then there was the Jabberwock.

She was there on Sunday morning: a white woman who looked to be in her forties, with glassy bright eyes, a shock of bleached blonde hair, and a manic belligerent energy. Name: Jackie. She'd been installed in the bookcase-adjacent bedroom, having arrived, I assume, late Saturday night. (Vaseline Man had been relocated to the sixth room—the one next to the nurses' station, the one I'd suspected was a padded cell but turned out to be just another ordinary twin-bed setup.) Jackie stayed in her room with the door barely ajar, not mingling at all, emerging only to grab meals and wolf them down. She talked to herself, spitting out the words like an irritated boss chastising a problematic employee. For the first 48 hours, she did not attend Group, but on Tuesday morning she emerged, wearing her disposable scrubs and grippy socks, and joined us—Counselor Paula, Reyes, Tessa, Albert, and me; Miranda the Gryphon was napping—at one of the round tea tables. She perched on the edge of a chair, her right leg jiggling.

Paula greeted her warmly: "Jackie, we're so glad to have you. Everyone, this is Jackie."

"Hi, Jackie," we chorused.

"Yeah, hi," said Jackie, her overbright eyes flicking to and fro.

"Let's all introduce ourselves," said Paula.

We did. Jackie gave her full name then said, in a pleasant-enough tone, "Yeah, nice to meet you all, but I can't stay here much longer. I hafta get back to my crime syndicate."

Thinking she was making a little joke, and quite a funny one at that, everyone (except Tessa, who of course hadn't heard) smiled and chuckled.

"No! I'm serious!" Her voice tensed. "I run a crime syndicate out of my home. It's a big deal, I have ten employees. Cashflow of fifteen, twenty grand a month. I have to be there to keep it running, the other guys can't do it, they're not competent, I can't trust them—"

Paula interjected: "All right, Jackie, that's fine, we can discuss that later. Now, let me explain a little bit about our routine here in the behavioral health ward."

Jackie fell silent and sat back in her chair, leg jiggling, eyes flicking.

"Breakfast," Paula continued, "is at seven. Then you can order your meals for the day and get dressed and have some free time. TV hours are 7:30 a.m. to 9:30 p.m.—or is it 10?"

"It's 10," I said, helpfully.

"Right, 10 p.m. So then, at 10 every morning, we have Group. Group is mandatory—"

"Wait—" Jackie sat bolt upright, frowning. "Are you *threatening* me?"

"What?" said Paula. "No, I just—"

"Yes you did, I heard you! You threatened me! If you're gonna threaten me, I'm gonna report you to the hospital board. I have connections on the hospital board. They will hear about this!" Jackie stood up, forefinger jabbing, six inches of bleached blonde hair sticking out around her taut, glaring face. Her voice rose to a shout. "You can*not* threaten me! That is *illegal*. I'm gonna file a report. You'll see, you're gonna be in *big* trouble!" We watched her wheel around and stomp off to her room, spitting curses.

> … the Jabberwock, with eyes of flame
> Came whiffling through the tulgey wood,
> And burbled as it came.

Kerfuffle over, we patients turned placidly back to the table, expecting Group to recommence. But Paula seemed shaken; with trembling hands she pulled her shawl tighter around her shoulders and said, "My goodness. I was only trying to explain the routine."

I felt sorry for the White Queen but sorrier for Jackie; she was obviously terrified, her Jabberwock act a mere front. Surely, I thought, a psych ward therapist would be used to this sort of minor freakout? The nurses clearly were. I looked at Paula and shook my head, trying to inject all-purpose sympathy into my expression. "She's not ready," I said.

"I didn't want to upset her! I was only trying to explain— to explain the routine." Paula was almost sniffling. The others around the table regarded her blankly.

I considered patting her shoulder, thought better of it, and repeated: "She's not ready."

Kind of nuts, I thought, that I'm the one offering reassurance, here. Isn't it supposed to be the other way round? On the other hand, it was nice to be in a position to offer reassurance. I hadn't been in that position for a long time.

———

Paula and I were having a one-on-one chat during recreation. "I've realized, Jocelyn," she said, "that when you look angry in Group, you're not really angry. You're just taking it all in."

Nah, I thought, I'm actually pretty angry. I just hide it better than the Jabberwock.

"But the good thing about you," she went on, "is that you always *try*."

True, I thought. When Matt yelled *you're not trying*, he was wrong: I was trying, just trying too many things and not sticking with any. But if White Queen Paula meant to imply that the other patients didn't try as hard as I did, she, too, was wrong. One lesson I took away from Madland is that as long as a person is doing anything at all—brushing their teeth, fetching a meal tray, coloring a picture, grunting "Good morning," talking about their crime syndicate—they *are* trying, maybe not in the same way as the next person, but trying nonetheless.

"Come, tell me how you live," says Lewis Carroll's traveler to the aged, aged man a-sitting on a gate, and when the aged man replies ("I look for butterflies ... I make them into mutton pies"), the traveler won't accept the answer. "Come, tell me how you live!" he shouts again and again while thumping the aged man on the head, and his target, undaunted and uncomplaining, offers a new answer each time: "I go my ways, and when I find a mountain rill, I set it in a blaze," which, he says, results in a substance called Rowland's Macassar Oil (something like Vaseline, perhaps?) that he sells for twopence halfpenny. Or "I hunt for haddocks' eyes among the heather bright ..." Or "I sometimes dig for buttered rolls, or set limed twigs for crabs ..." The aged man knows many odd methods for making a living, and he just keeps putting them out there, doggedly, until the traveler finally hears and thanks him. And now, says the traveler,

> ... if e'er by chance I put
> My fingers into glue,
> Or madly squeeze a right-hand foot
> Into a left-hand shoe,
> Or if I drop upon my toe
> A very heavy weight,
> I weep, for it reminds me so
> Of that old man I used to know—
> Whose look was mild, whose speech was slow,
> Whose hair was whiter than the snow,
> Whose face was very like a crow,
> With eyes, like cinders, all aglow,
> Who seemed distracted with his woe,
> Who rocked his body to and fro,
> And muttered mumblingly and low,
> As if his mouth were full of dough,

Who snorted like a buffalo—
That summer evening, long ago,
A-sitting on a gate.

Most Madlanders seem distracted with their woe; many rock their body to and fro as they mutter mumblingly; some even snort like a buffalo, with eyes like cinders all aglow, scaring well-meaning therapists who tell them Group is mandatory. We can acknowledge that some of the mentally ill can't be trusted in society and must be contained, while still acknowledging this: Every last one of them is trying, trying however they are able.

Nowadays, when I find myself struggling with gluey projects or wrong-footed decisions or weighty misfortunes, the cluttered mucky obstacle course that is human life, I think of those men and women—young and old, cheerful and woeful—who were confined with me in the St. Giles psych ward in the first two weeks of November 2020. Most of us got better and got out. One or two of us didn't, but it wasn't for lack of trying.

————

The Jabberwock incident happened on Tuesday, the day before I was to be discharged. Let's backtrack now to the evening of Saturday, November fourteenth, the ides of November, nearly four months since the storm demons had invited themselves into my brain and announced their intention to stay. Since that announcement, I had logged four weeks of stoicism in the face of an upsetting but tolerable disruption; four weeks of focused, rational efforts to evict the intruders by means of medicines, therapies, and attitude adjustments; three weeks of increasingly grinding, sleepless desperation, culminating with the decampment to the healing center only to find that the devilish revelers had followed me there undeterred; and finally, three weeks of a white-knuckle nosedive into hell while the demons, now become my landlords, rocked and rolled and poked me with their pitchforks, 22 hours of every goddamned day.

Things now were much improved. I knew this because during my most recent team meeting (this one presided over by Dr. Denali, the hospital's chief psychiatrist and a most impressive female Caterpillar, whose tone when she said, "Let's make it a great day" made clear that it wasn't a suggestion), I had turned to Nurse Annette and asked, "Do *you* think I'm getting better?" She smiled broadly and nodded yes. I chose to believe her. Plus I had the mantra given me by Dr. Taylor: *You will know. You will know. When it happens, you will know.*

And yet ... although the vertigo chop had subsided, the anxiety tides had ebbed, and I'd been achieving my stated goal of six hours' sleep per night, a clutch of demon diehards still remained: committed to a party that had dragged on too long, reaching that stage where the house reeks of cigarette butts doused in beer and a bleary pothead, off in a corner, is head-banging to Pink Floyd's "The Wall" as a dismal dawn creeps through the windows. I felt stuck in a mental hangover, trapped in an emotional ashtray. While I was more or less functional—and hooray for that—it seemed unlikely I'd ever feel *happy* again. Happiness would take a miracle, I thought, and sorry, Miranda, but I don't believe God is in the miracle business these days.

At 8:10 p.m., the ward was unusually quiet. Bonnie, in Room 1, had retired for the night; Miranda and Reyes, in Room 3, were preparing for bed; Albert, who'd been ambling around the dayroom peeking in bedroom doorways as if hoping to be invited in for a cozy chat, was told by Nurse Yvonne to cut it out and had retreated, obedient, to his own room; and Tessa was huddled on one of the side couches, her long hair damp from a shower, reading a paperback. Nurse Wendy was the other nurse on duty tonight; she would be off again, I knew, tomorrow through Tuesday, but for tonight I was in her charge and feeling relatively secure in her cheerful ingénue presence and Yvonne's matronly one. I had put on my pajamas and finished coloring my flowers-and-leaves page. Now I was at loose ends.

The TV was off—again, unusual for this early hour—but hey, who was queen of the remote? Me! I shuffled over, clicked the power button, and flipped through a few channels. Oh look, I thought, it's *27 Dresses*. Same damn movies on every night, just like in the real world. Looks to be about a third of the way in, that's too bad; not as if I don't know the plot, though, might as well stick with it. I leaned back and watched Katherine Heigl in a hideous olive-green bridesmaid dress telling Weddings Reporter Guy that she was "a very good caulker," nudge nudge wink wink. Then a rumbling sound alerted me to the snack cart (*bit late tonight, eh?*) being pushed in by Nurse Yvonne. "Snacks are here," she announced quietly to the air. I got up and went to look. The healthy selections seemed limited this evening: a brown-spotted banana, a tough-skinned apple, Jell-o but no pudding, the usual juice cups, a lone granola bar. I was thinking glumly that I'd have to fall back on one of the nutrition drinks prescribed me by the hospital dietician, now sitting unopened in a vitamin-rich but cloying array on my credenza, when my eye fell on a largeish bag of ... Fritos.

A dialogue ensued.

> **Mad Me:** I can't have those. Fritos are junk food.
>
> **Sane Me:** *Yeah. They look kinda good, though, don't they?*
>
> **Mad Me:** They do, kind of, but I really shouldn't have any.
>
> **Sane Me:** *Why not? What'll happen if you eat a bag of Fritos?*
>
> **Mad Me:** I dunno ... probably ... like ...
>
> **Sane Me:** *I'll tell ya what: nothing.*

Mad Me: Nothing? Really? You think?

Sane Me: *Yup. Nothing.*

Mad Me: Hmm. I guess I could have some milk with them. Balance them out.

Sane Me: *You could. Look, there's a little carton of milk right there.*

Mad Me: Fritos and milk, wow. That sounds …

Sane Me: *Tasty?*

Mad Me: Well … yes.

Sane Me: *When it happens, you will know.*

Mad Me:

Sane Me: *When it happens—*

Mad Me: —I will know! Yes! I will eat these Fritos, yes I said *yes I will yes!*

I grabbed milk carton and chip bag, returned to the TV couch, plopped down, squeezed open the carton spout and tore open the top of the bag without difficulty. I leaned back, propping my right ankle on my left knee. Then for the next hour I lounged comfortably, by myself, chortling now and then at the galumphing romantic antics of Katherine Heigl and Weddings Reporter Guy, sipping the cool sweet milk, munching the salty crunchy Fritos.

I ate the whole bag. I felt happy. And I thanked all the gods, because it was a miracle.

PART IV

The Door in the Wall

CHAPTER 11

IT'S MY OWN INVENTION

I'm sitting at the dining-room table in a regular chair—haven't used the rocking chair in months—sipping mint tea and reading yet another newspaper article about the Covid vaccines: who's getting them, who isn't, do they work, what about side effects. I got mine in April, the Johnson & Johnson single jab, administered by a nice young Army soldier who wasn't nearly as good with a needle as Oscar the pharmacist, but still, much appreciated, and so far I guess it's working because I'm feeling pretty good. This summer of 2021 has been surprisingly cool; Matt and I haven't even felt the need to hold our traditional discussion about how we must, really must, put in air conditioning this year. Right now Matt is in his basement office, sending up a thunk-thunk-thunk of vigorous one-fingered typing through the delightfully nonbouncy floor. As I take another sip of tea, my phone buzzes. It's a notification from the Mayo Clinic.

Having left the ward on November eighteenth and made it through the holidays, and with a steady regimen of meds and a strict sleep schedule (eleven to seven, no excuses) doing their job, I turned my attention once again to acquiring a diagnosis, or at least an explanation, for what had happened. I was not looking forward to another round of groveling for doctors' appointments, but turns out, when you've been in the madhouse, doctors take your calls. I managed to see both Dr. Ortega and Dr. Greene in person, and I had phone sessions monthly with psychiatrist Dr. Funar, weekly with therapist Denise. In February, I finally got a VNG test: that same test I was prescribed long ago by the Queen of Hearts but never underwent, the one where they put you in goggles, flash sparkly lights in your eyes, and puff hot and cold air (not water, water it turns out is old fashioned) in your ears. The procedure was no big deal, and the results, according to Dr. Greene when I saw him for follow-up, were normal.

"What does *normal* mean, in this case?" I asked.

"It means there's no imbalance in your ears," Dr. Greene said, peering into his computer screen as he rubbed the dome of his egglike head. "No damage to either side. Normal."

"Oh. What if there's damage to *both* sides?"

"Mm. No. That's not how it works. The results show your ears are perfectly balanced, so there's no damage. It has to be a central issue, in the brain. Something an MRI would pick up."

"But I thought my MRI was normal, too."

"Yep. At this point, I would suggest you see a neurologist. I'll give you three referrals."

One of the referrals was to Dr. Andersen, the "green, Denver, horse" guy who had demanded to know *why* I couldn't sleep and pronounced me a migraine sufferer. The other two doctors, per Google, had retired or moved away. It was time, I figured, to consult a real expert, and without further ado I booked an appointment with Adele, my beloved longtime hair stylist. She'd reopened her salon in March: one customer at a time, masks required.

"You should go to the Mayo," Adele said, snipping my no-longer-dyed, completely white hair into a refreshing pixie cut. "All my clients with weird diseases go to the Mayo. Nobody bothers with the specialists in Santa Fe. Lift your mask loops."

I lifted the loops so she could snip around my ears, making sure to hold the cloth over my nose and mouth. "I don't know if I can get in," I said. "The Mayo doesn't take just anyone."

"They'll take you. Tilt your head down for me … They like the weird brain things."

I phoned the Mayo Scottsdale. The screener wasn't impressed by my reports of an odd type of vertigo, but when I made a quick pivot to *undiagnosed neurological disorder with multiple symptoms that caused suicidal ideation and landed me in the hospital for two weeks*, she perked up and got me an appointment with Dr. Goodman, chief of Neurology, for June 21st. "Complete all the questionnaires and submit all your medical records through the portal," she said. "And make sure you can stay for at least four days, because there will be a lot of tests."

Excellent, I thought, I want all the tests, every single one. I clicked up the Southwest Airlines website and booked a round-trip ticket to Phoenix for the third week of June.

——————

The 102-degree Arizona heat painted my skin as I made the short walk from the Mayo campus hotel—a La Quinta, I think it was—to the clinic. I was wearing a sleeveless white-and-purple flowered dress, white cotton blazer, chic purple flats, gold jewelry. (Alert, cooperative, well-groomed!) The time was 10:30 a.m., miles too early for my noon appointment with Dr. Goodman, but I planned to hang out for a while and get the lay of the land; I was sure there'd be food on offer somewhere, and indeed, after checking in at the main desk on the first floor, checking in again at the Neurology desk on the second floor, filling out another sheaf of forms, and receiving my "no Covid" handstamp, the receptionist said I was welcome to visit the café on the ground level as long as I came back in good time. I went back to the elevators and down. The facility was huge, well appointed, and eerily hushed, like something out of a post-apocalyptic novel. As I walked along, I passed spacious waiting lounges, lush displays of greenery around trickling fountains, and arrowed signs suspended from the ceiling, pointing the way to dozens of destinations: Cardiology, Pulmonology, Otolaryngology, Endocrinology,

Restrooms, Parking, Oncology, Business Office, Restrooms. The carpet throughout was brown sprinkled with mid-century modern circles of blue and yellow. Sanitizer stations and "Facemasks Required" placards were plentiful; human beings were few.

After a snack in the nearly empty café, I returned to Neurology and took a seat in the waiting area beside a wall of shrubbery. I scrolled through social media posts, then texted with Susan. "You've named all the plants by now, haven't you?" she wrote. "Hahaha yep," I replied. Eight or ten other patients were seated in the rows of leatherette chairs, and there were long intervals between summonses. As my phone displayed 12:01, then 12:08, then 12:17, I started to worry that they'd changed their minds and decided not to see me: maybe my weird brain thing wasn't weird enough for them after all. But at 12:20, a tech emerged from the inner sanctum, nose to his electronic tablet, and called out, "Joyce, uh, Joycelyn Davis?"

To my surprise, there was no pre-interview; the tech merely confirmed my basic information and ushered me straight into an office. I settled myself for another long wait, but a moment later the door opened and in came the chief himself: tall, white-coated, bespectacled, exuding affable expertise. He looked like a TV doctor.

"Hello, Ms. Davis, I'm Dr. Goodman, it's very nice to meet you," he said, extending his hand for a casual-yet-professional shake. "So sorry to keep you waiting. We try hard to keep on schedule, but I'm afraid we've been running behind today."

Wow! I thought. Giving him ten out of ten for his entrance.

By the end of the session, however, his score had dropped. Oh, he took plenty of time: nearly a full hour. And he listened with good eye contact and an intelligent air of interest. But for all that, he was a Caterpillar—a Caterpillar Supreme, in fact. Here's a sampling of our exchanges, along with his declining ratings as I posted them to my mental scoreboard:

He: "Says here you're an author. What kind of books do you write?"

Me: "Business books, mostly. About leadership, strategy, things like that. I used to be an executive at a consulting firm."

He: (looking bemused) "Really? Huh. And do you enjoy that? Writing books, I mean."

Rating: 9.5

He: "OK, so ..." (riffling through a stack of print-outs that includes my medical records and completed questionnaires, submitted to the portal months ago as instructed) "... I see I have your very *long* explanation, here. Gosh, it's almost a book! Tell me about this book of yours, ha-ha!"

Me: "Ha-ha, sure. Do you want the whole story?"

He: "I guess. Well, no, just gimme the headlines."

Rating: 8.7

Me: "... so, according to the VNG, my inner ears are normal."

He: (looking at the VNG report from Dr. Greene's office) "But it says here, abnormal."

Me: "What?"

He: "See?" (pointing to the paper, which I can't see) "It says *abnormal*."

Me: "That's odd. Dr. Greene told me my ears were totally normal. He said there was no imbalance, no damage, and I needed to see a neurologist. That's definitely what he said."

He: "Well, I'm just saying, that's what it says here. Abnormal."

Rating: 7.9

He: (looking at my MRI images on his computer screen) "These images are very low quality."

Me: "Yeah, doesn't surprise me. It was an upright machine, and I think it was pretty old."

He: (pointing) "Look, see how low quality it is? I haven't seen one like this since the 1990s. I mean, it's basically worthless."

Me: (nodding, without the least idea what I'm looking at) "Yep, I see what you mean. Low quality. Uh-huh."

Rating: 7.4

He: "… and I'm going to order you two different neuropathy tests. I can tell you right now that the one for the long nerves, where they zap you with electrodes, is going to come back fine, but I'm most interested in the one for the small nerves. It's a skin punch, about yay big" (holding up thumb and forefinger a quarter inch apart). "They'll take two punches from your leg, then we analyze the skin to see if there's anything wrong. I'm also ordering you another MRI, so we can get a real look at your brain, and a whole set of blood tests. We'll check for everything: MS, cancer, diabetes, autoimmune, everything. But my bet at this point is on the small fiber neuropathy. How does that sound? Any questions?"

Me: (realizing we're at the end) "Thanks, that makes sense about the neuropathy causing the pain and itching, but I guess my question is, um, what do you think was up with the vertigo? And why such a major mental collapse? I mean, I was locked in a psych ward, for gosh sake!"

He: (with a wave of the hand) "Meh ... You just got in funk."

You just got in a funk? With that, his rating plummeted to a flat six. Maybe even a five.

———

That afternoon, I went first to the business office to deal with insurance matters, then to the lab where I had an appointment for blood drawing. The clearly super-competent tech took six vials in rapid succession, pausing only to ask, "You doin' OK?" I was. I walked back to the hotel in the frying heat, bought some dinner from the food bar (selections limited because Covid, but eatable), watched a couple episodes of *Grey's Anatomy* on my Kindle, and went to bed.

Next day, Tuesday, I had the neuropathy tests. The first one, to test my long nerves, was quite painful: I lay on an exam table and a nurse used a zapper to zap me in a dozen places on my arms and legs, each zap lasting about three seconds, while another nurse observed a computer screen with squiggly green lines representing (I suppose) my reflexes. Later I returned for the second test, the skin biopsy, which wasn't so bad: they numbed me up and excised two round, pencil-eraser-sized chunks of flesh, one from my left calf, one from my left thigh. I felt almost nothing. The highlight of that session, though, was the very smart nurse who ran it. She was, she said, a Master of Science in nursing, and before doing the skin punches she sat me in a chair and gave me a vivid, detailed explanation of small fiber neuropathy. It went something like this:

> You've got your big nerves, or long fibers, running along your muscles, and then you've got your millions of tiny nerves, or small fibers, which form a network all over your body, like tiny twigs branching off a tree. Sometimes, some of those tiny nerves die off or get damaged. And since it's a network, if some nerves go missing, the remaining nerves can't send their signals too well, and they misfire. It's like when a few bulbs on a string of lights burn out and the rest of the bulbs start flickering. When your tiny nerves are misfiring like that, you can get patches of burning, itching, or tingling. That's small fiber neuropathy.

"I see!" I said, drinking in the coherence. "And do we know what causes it?"

"There are hundreds of possible causes. Diabetes is one of the most common ones, also autoimmune diseases, but 50 percent of the time we don't know the cause. It's idiopathic." Her tone was informational, adult to adult. "But the good news is, we can diagnose it: we do the skin punches, we measure the density of the nerve fibers in those bits of skin, and if the density is less than normal, we know for sure you've got it."

There was a young doctor in the room, sitting to one side; Smart Nurse had introduced him as "Dr. _____, a resident in training" and asked if I minded him observing. "Not at all," I'd said. Now I turned to this resident, pointed at Smart Nurse, and remarked, "She's really good."

He agreed, nodding.

Smart Nurse smiled through her facemask. "It's all about patient education! I tell everyone, education is everything. We have to take the time to educate. OK, ready to do this?"

I stretched out on the exam table, thinking, I wish more doctors would take a page from you, Smart Nurse. *One also notes* (Sane Me remarked pointedly) *that you never did have shingles.*

Next came the MRI, scheduled for Wednesday at six p.m. MRIs, it transpired, were performed not at the clinic but at the Mayo Hospital, which is in downtown Phoenix. I rode the shuttle bus there along with a motley crew of Fellow Sicklings, arriving, again, far too early. I set up camp in the cafeteria; not nearly as nice as the clinic café, but I bought a tuna wrap, potato chips, and a vitamin water and ate at a table beside an enormous tinted window that stood up gamely to the halogen glare of the evening sun. As I ate I stared, fascinated, at an airport-style digital announcement board displaying a long list of partial patient names, ID numbers, and color-coded progress indicators: "Prepping," "In Surgery," "Waking Up," "Ready for Visitors." As I like to do in airports, I imagined, ghoulishly, what would be posted in the event of a disaster. "Delayed," maybe? Better than "Never Waking Up."

I'd already checked in and filled out forms, so when I re-presented myself in the Radiology department at 5:55 p.m. there was only a short wait before a tech ushered me back to a spotless staging area furnished with armchairs, lockers, and changing cubicles all done in soft beiges and blues. She gave me a locker key, a cotton gown that was almost my size, and a pair of gray grippy socks adorned with the requisite smiley faces. "You can change in there and put your belongings in a locker," she said. "Oh, and you're welcome to keep the socks."

I don't know if it was the clonazepam, the Zoloft, or simply that going to hell and back inures one to minor medical trials, but I sailed through that second MRI with barely a blink. The machine was brightly lit, wide enough, open on both ends, and not that long. When they slid me in, I could look down and see my hips and legs still outside the tube. The first part took only fifteen minutes, then they slid me out, injected the contrast dye, and slid me in to bake for another five. No television was on offer, but it didn't matter, for the air of expensive, whirring efficiency was far more soothing than the Property Brothers could ever be. Once done, I returned to the staging area to shed the gown and resume my clothes. I kept the socks.*

At home over the next two weeks, my results trickled in on the patient portal. Blood tests: normal. Zap test: normal. MRI: normal. Although Dr. You-Just-Got-in-a-Funk had ordered another goggles and lights test, I'd been unable to schedule it before leaving Scottsdale. Judging from the suppressed rage on the face of the Neurology scheduler as she talked down the phone to the Otolaryngology scheduler, Mayo Brains and Mayo Ears didn't exactly get along, and Mayo Ears wasn't inclined to fit me in on such discourteously short notice. (Never mind, I thought, I could track down Dr. Greene and make him re-explain my normal-abnormal VNG.) As the second week of July rolled in, the only outstanding item was the small fiber neuropathy test. I was fully expecting that one to come back normal, too. What a colossal waste of time, I thought, sipping my mint tea at the dining room table. I might as well have stayed in Santa Fe.

Then I heard my phone buzz. I tapped the Mayo icon, logged in to the portal, and clicked through to find a message from a nurse assistant. It read as follows:

> Thank you for your use of the patient portal. Dr. Goodman has reviewed the results of your recent testing. Please be aware of the following:

---

* Back home and in receipt of the Mayo's co-pay bill, I dubbed these socks my Eight Hundred Dollar Grippy Socks and the ones from the psych ward my Free Grippy Socks. To be fair, the latter are ankle length and flimsy, while the ones from the Mayo reach to the knee and still haven't worn through. Eight hundred did seem a little excessive for socks, though.

Please inform the patient that we received her epidermal skin biopsy and it did show the biopsy from her left calf with significantly reduced nerve fiber density consistent with a small fiber neuropathy as we suspected. We now have a diagnosis of small fiber neuropathy to explain her paresthesias and dysesthesias so we have an answer to what is causing her symptoms. Thank you

"Hey! Oh my god, hey, hey, look at this!" Clutching the phone, I got up and raced downstairs to Matt's office to tell him the news: "It's a diagnosis! This is what's wrong with me! I HAVE A DIAGNOSIS!"

And with diagnosis in the bag, I could finally piece together a solution to the mystery. I offer that solution now, with all the usual caveats: I am not a doctor, this isn't intended as medical advice, consult your own healthcare provider, and so forth. What happened to me is what happened to me, and to me alone. I call it the Perfect Storm.

It was a typhoon in the brain, that storm, the result of four lesser tempests which, over the course of roughly a decade, arrived in this order: 1) perimenopause, 2) small fiber neuropathy, 3) mal debarquement vertigo, and (maybe) 4) a mild case of Covid. I see a causation arrow from the first to the second to the third; the fourth, I suspect, was just a random interloper. Once these tempests got going, however, they fed off one another, gaining force and spinning off more squalls—insomnia, anxiety, sound sensitivity, eyesight issues, breathing problems—which fed back into the original four, and soon I was caught in a self-sustaining all-pervading mind-body maelstrom, with no way to calm it except to "shut it down," as Dr. Ortega said later. "What you have to do in these cases," she said, "is just shut the brain down, allow it to rest, then as long as there're no deep structural issues, it will often heal itself." I was reminded, when she said that, of the last-resort treatment used by country vet James Herriott (*All Creatures Great and Small*) on sick animals trapped in a harrowing loop of fever, thirst, drinking, retching, more fever, more thirst, more drinking … He'd inject an anesthetic in a nearly lethal dose, putting the sheep or dog into a 48-hour coma in which it could have absolute rest, rest without fear, pain, or strain. A factory reset, if you will. Thankfully, I didn't need a reset that drastic or risky; I did, however, need a hospital stay with two weeks of medicated shutdown. And I did heal.

But how did the storm get started in the first place?

It started with menopause. This entire book could have been written as a menopause story, since perimenopause* was the ongoing condition that frayed my nerves and set the stage for the subsequent drama. When I asked Dr. Ortega if she had seen this type of near-total mental collapse followed by near-complete recovery before, she said, "Yes, I see it fairly often in teenage girls and middle-aged women. The hormonal fluctuations of puberty and perimenopause can put the brain chemically on edge, and then anything might trigger a meltdown: a virus, bacterial infection, emotional trauma …"

"Or vertigo?" I asked, fascinated by this new information.

"Yes, absolutely! In your case, I guess vertigo was the trigger."

It made sense. I'd had a rocky time with hormones ever since my teen years, experiencing anxiety, panic attacks, depression, and sleep disturbances in seven- to ten-day waves linked to my very irregular menstrual cycle. When I hit a still-more-rocky

---

* Perimenopause, the period surrounding menopause (the cessation of menstruation), can last anywhere from a few years to decades. Some of us hit it in our late 30s, and it can continue into our 60s. When people talk of "a rough menopause," they're really talking about perimenopause and the myriad unpleasant symptoms that can accompany it. *Screaming to Be Heard*, by Dr. Elizabeth Vliet, is one of the best sources I've found on the topic.

perimenopause at age 40 and my doctor put me on a regimen of birth control pills, I thought I'd found the solution, and when I shifted to estradiol pills upon hitting actual menopause at age 51, then the patch at 55, I assumed that same solution would keep on working. I didn't realize that even when you supplement your natural hormones with exogenous ones, the natural hormones continue to party on, careless of the steadying influences you have introduced, still capable of wreaking havoc. In the weeks before the vertigo's big return on July 16, 2020, I'd experienced night sweats, odd visual phenomena, and a marked deepening of the voice, all of which are menopausal symptoms and all of which I ignored, confident that my faithful estradiol patch—albeit at a very low dose by then—was taking care of me. And no doubt it was, to an extent. But a low-dose hormone patch, I have learned, is no match for an anxiety disorder whipped up by hormones gone wild.

Perimenopause, then, gave me a distressed brain, teetering on a ledge, susceptible to anything that cared to come along and give it a good hard shove. The principal shover, in my case, was the vertigo. But what led to the vertigo?

"So, I guess the small fiber neuropathy was responsible." I was at the dining table again, shouting into Zoom on a hot August afternoon. The Mayo neurology resident's smiling face filled the screen. Dr. You-Just-Got-In-a-Funk was there, too, in the side video box; he appeared distracted and was letting his subordinate take the lead in this follow-up appointment.

"The neuropathy attacked my ears, right? And that caused the mal debarquement?"

"No, no," Smiling Resident said. "Small fiber neuropathy is peripheral, not central. It can't cause vertigo. No, no."

"But the inner ears *are* peripheral," I said. "I mean, they're not in the brain or the spinal cord. So they're peripheral. And if they're damaged ..."

"Uhh, no. *Peripheral* is, like, your arms and legs." Smiling Resident smiled even more broadly as Dr. In-a-Funk shuffled papers, paying no attention. "Neuropathy doesn't cause vertigo. Now, how would you describe your pain level today?"

"It's fine. Little area on my left arm acting up, but it's fine."

I stifled a sigh. According to Dr. Greene, my ears were normal, so the problem must be my abnormal brain. According to both MRI scans, my brain was normal, so the problem must be my abnormal ears. And now, according to the Mayo people, my peripheral nerves were abnormal, but my ears weren't included in that abnormal periphery. Ears, evidently, were a no-man's land, neither central nor peripheral, under the purview of ENTs, not neurologists. And my ENT had said my ears were normal—even though the report sent by his office had said abnormal. It was all very confusing. But never mind; to me, the owner of the ears, brain, and nerves in question, the answer had become pretty clear.

Inner-ear nerves, I reasoned, are indeed peripheral—for ears are peripheral organs, not part of the brain or spinal cord—and mine were, how shall I put it? Messed up. Over the years, the raw burning neuropathy had attacked, among other places, the left side of my head and left ear, then the right side and right ear, each attack lasting two or three weeks, each one foreshadowing a spinning episode which quickly resolved into mal debarquement vertigo plus a dizzy inability to lie on one side. Because the attacks had occurred equally on both left and right, Dr. Greene was correct: there was no imbalance. And because it was *small fiber* neuropathy, neither was there any major nerve damage: no harm to the big vestibular nerves, just a thinning of the tiny dendrites, like an old t-shirt grown threadbare in the wash or a net of holiday lights with a few dead bulbs. Those thinned-out nerves were now wont to "misfire" (as Smart Nurse had put it), causing staticky signals to be sent to my vestibular nerve and hence to my brain, signals ever so slightly out of sync with what my eyes and body were reporting.*

What's a brain to do, when confronted with ears saying one thing and eyes/body saying another? Well, at first it's liable to freak out: *What the fuck is this!? Eyes and body say world is stable, ears say world is moving ... something is terribly wrong I'm sick I'm dizzy I'm spinning I'm falling helllp!!* But if it's clever (and all human brains are very clever indeed), it will immediately start to work out the problem, thus:

> Hang on, hang on, let's not panic. Think: where have we experienced this before? Think think think ... Oh! I know! This is just like when we're riding in a plane, or a train, or below decks in a boat. Our body doesn't *feel* like it's moving, and the floor doesn't *look* like it's moving, yet our inner ears say: "Moving!" These mixed signals are called—wait, wait, don't tell me, I know this one—*being in a state of passive motion.*

> We actually started our whole life this way, didn't we? Rocking along inside mom's womb, bouncy, bouncy, safe and secure. Cool. I know what the deal is now, and there's no need to worry, because I, The Brain, shall interpret this situation for you.

> You're on a boat—yeah, that's it, a boat. Or a plane, or a train, whatever. Let's call it a boat. The ground is bouncing and swaying, but you don't need to feel sick, because boats are normal, you know all about boats. You can balance, because you've got your sea legs. And now you can stop freaking out and go on with your life. You're welcome!

---

* According to Dr. Greene, frayed nerve fibers also tend to release those wicked little calcium crystals (otochonia) into the ear canals. So it's possible the Knave of Hearts was right again: I perhaps *had* had BPPV, which spun me around then resolved on its own, leaving me with just the misfiring nerves ... and mal debarquement.

... Eh? What's that? You don't *like* the bouncy-rocky boat feeling?

OK then, would you prefer we go back to that crazy dizzy sick sensation where you can't stand up and you want to scream and barf? No? Didn't think so. Now shut up and go make us a drink. I'ma enjoy this boat ride!

Dear, sweet, atavistic brain. It works all that out in a matter of seconds, then dusts off its hands and moves on to more pressing matters, such as managing digestion, osmosing oxygen, and scanning the vicinity for signs of impending doom. Problem is, with its masterful interpretation of screwy ear signals as "state of passive motion," the brain has inadvertently created a *new* sign of impending doom: a perpetual turbulence of the earth, featuring loopy lurches, disorienting drops, and jostling jounces that persist all day, all night, ceaseless, terrifying. The brain doesn't like it any more than you do, but it knows there's a choice: walk on water, or don't walk at all. It chooses the former, because its priority is to keep you alive, and when it comes to staying alive, being able to walk is really helpful. The disadvantages of a turbulent earth are significant but, in the brain's view, are outweighed by the advantages.

"Relax, I'll keep you safe," says the brain, jotting a note not to let you sleep too deeply until this bouncy ground situation has been resolved. "Here, I'll crank up the adrenaline. Can't be too careful. But don't worry, I'm on the case! I won't let you die."

Thanks, Brain.

I don't know why my brain seized on Boat World as the solution. Mal de Débarquement Syndrome is rare, while vertigo attacks in general are not rare at all, so it seems only a few brains react the way mine did. What I do know is that the main sufferers from MdDS are women aged 40 to 60; that is, perimenopausal women. And I know that perimenopause can throw the whole nervous system, central and peripheral, into a state of frazzlement. Putting it all together, I conclude that perimenopause led to the small fiber neuropathy, small fiber neuropathy led to the vertigo, my anxious-but-clever brain dealt with the vertigo by inventing Boat World, and then came … Covid?

This is the puzzle piece of which I am most unsure. In the summer of 2020, the pandemic was raging across New Mexico, the vaccines were still nine months away, and although most Santa Feans did mask up and stay home, we were never in full lockdown. In the weeks after the vertigo struck, I remember another strange symptom: an apnea-like closing of the throat that would cause me to jerk awake with a gasp, multiple times, just as I was falling asleep. I think this apnea gasp, added to the discomforts of Boat World, was what flipped the No Sleep switch. Clever Brain was being clever again: If the earth has turned to water *and* you can't breathe, it's best not to sleep at all, for nodding off, even briefly, might mean drowning, suffocating, or both. No wonder I was pathologically alert, my mind and senses tuned to mortal danger.

Was the apnea the result of a mild case of coronavirus, contracted in mid-July and concluded long before mid-October when I entered the True Healing Center and got my first Q-tip up the nose? I don't remember any other viral symptoms, except—well, I did have a *very* hoarse voice for a while, there. And often when I woke in the night, I'd feel a heaviness in my chest, a shortness of breath, which worsened if I rolled onto my back. And those night sweats I'd had in mid-July: were they perhaps the result of a fever, not hormonal swings?

I can't be sure. Covid tests weren't readily available then, and anyway my particular symptoms didn't seem to call for one. In those first six weeks of my Madland journey, I was chalking everything up to hormones and "my bizarre boat thing." All I can say is that, in hindsight, it seems more likely than not that Covid was in the mix.[*]

Finally, a word on the medical treatments. Most of them—from acyclovir to acupuncture, Ambien to Seroquel, thunder shirts to Epley maneuvers—were useless or worse than useless. Here are the three meds that ended up helping me, plus my thoughts on why they did.

Zoloft (sertraline). "When it works you will know," said Dr. Taylor, and he was right: it did work, and I did know. It took, however, a solid month to work, and I've since learned that an SSRI's positive effects often do take a month or more to weigh in, despite the standard line of "it might take a week or two." Why so long? One theory is that while these medications probably cause a short-term increase in the amount of happy-chemical serotonin floating around in your skull, and this increase can make some folks feel better almost at once, the biggest benefits of SSRIs occur long term: they rewire your brain, helping it become more adaptable and resilient—a lush, green, cushiony lawn as opposed to a thin, patchy, brittle one. And full rewiring takes months, even years. Another difficulty with SSRIs is that they make many people feel worse (in some cases a *lot* worse) before they feel better. I don't know why this is, but I suspect it's because neurological rewiring isn't a painless process. There must have to be demolition before renovation, pruning before growth, all of which is bound to be a shock, perhaps violent enough to make Security Brain crank up the sirens. Which brings us to …

---

[*] What about shingles, stemming from the herpes zoster virus? Nope, I was utterly wrong about that. A couple years later I got a titer test for chickenpox, which is caused by the same virus; turns out I'd never had it. If you've never had chickenpox, you can't get shingles. Those hundreds of blue-striped acyclovir capsules were all for naught.

Klonopin (clonazepam). For me, these little pink pills served two purposes. First, though they didn't shut off the sirens entirely, they dialed the volume way down, granting me respite from the constant, shrieking anxiety and letting my brain rest and heal. Second, they reduced the mal debarquement vertigo. This might seem counterintuitive, for Valium and its sister drugs can also *cause* dizziness, but as Dr. In-a-Funk explained, benzos dampen signals going from the sensory organs to the brain. "The clonazepam," he said, "is muffling the noise from your ears." Thanks to this signal-dampening effect, any benzo will, I imagine, calm any type of vertigo; clonazepam, however, is particularly long-lasting, with no abrupt kick ("smooth" as Nurse Craig put it). That long, smooth action is just what a rocking, rolling brain needs in order to find its way back to a steady state. And speaking of rock and roll …

Hormones. Ah, those dedicated partiers, estrogen and progesterone, still dancing at the disco long after closing time. Like I said, an estradiol patch is no match for one's own natural disco inferno when it's really blazing. Still, I'd had the right idea when I asked Nurse Just-a-Nervous-Girl to adjust my patch dose upward, and I was right to ignore her scolding about "chasing the hormones." Most perimenopause symptoms are the result of a woman's brain and body having to adjust to much, much lower levels of estrogen than she has had since childhood; moreover, the hormonal decline isn't a sedate tram ride down a hill, but a rollercoaster ride down a mountain. A medication to ease that wild plunging descent, even a little, is for some women (like me) necessary. As for progesterone, I was also right when I told Dr. Greene that oral progesterone, when metabolized, releases a chemical similar to a benzo, which makes it helpful not only for sleep but also for dampening ear-to-brain signals. Again, none of these musings should be regarded as medical advice; that said,

I like to think of estrogen as a sort of natural Zoloft, progester-one as a sort of natural Klonopin.

So: the perfect storm. Perimenopause leads to neuropathy. Neuropathy leads to funny ear signals, hence vertigo. Brain deals with vertigo by inventing Boat World and, egged on by under-lying anxiety disorder, gets frightened by its own invention and decides Sleep Is Bad. The wind and waves rise, creeping up the shoreline, battering the piers and boardwalks, surging over the levees, feeding off their own energy, heedless of the sandbags and sheets of plywood being stacked or nailed by the humans in their path. And just as the whole weather system is feeling weary and thinking maybe it'll head out to sea and die down, here comes the Rona, swooping in to give it the extra punch it needs to become a Cat 5 hurricane.

————

Or, if you prefer cozy mysteries:
    Miss Firing Nerves
    Did it in the hormonal wreck room
    With the viral, vertiginous wrench.

CHAPTER 12

IN THE GOLDEN AFTERNOON

In the psych ward on Sunday morning, the morning after I ate the Fritos, I announced that I was feeling better and suggested I might go home soon. Everyone around the conference table—me, Nurse Annette, Red Queen Nadine, Dr. Taylor, and a random nursing student who was observing that day—looked at Chief Psychiatrist Denali and waited. Dr. Denali peered at me over her reading glasses, paused, looked down at her notepad while tapping her pen, paused, stared at the wall as the water and ice machine made an ice-making noise, peered at me again, then said, with slow deliberation:

"Mm hmm. Yes. I'm thinking … Wednesday."

The words of a Caterpillar are law. I knew right away that Wednesday would be my discharge day, not a day sooner or later, and that no one, neither nurse nor counselor nor junior doctor, would question or gainsay the decision.

The next 72 hours were action packed. Jacki the Jabberwock had arrived and was injecting a frisson of mafioso energy into the ward's routine even as she stayed sequestered in her room all day, muttering darkly about criminal schemes. Albert the Vaseline Man was vibing: watching TV, spreading cheer, occasionally unable to resist dropping some knowledge about Jesus Christ or petroleum jelly. Bonnie, though still clearly in low spirits, was out of her wheelchair most of the time, perambulating with the aid of a walker and eating regular meals. Reyes did yoga in the

241

sunroom whenever it was open. Miranda was making progress on getting into Casa Rosa, the group home; she spent a lot of time conferring with her social worker, often taking the phone to her room, which technically wasn't allowed, but turns out in Madland you can get away with many things that technically aren't allowed as long as you observe kindergarten rules: share nicely, use your words, be quiet during quiet time, keep your hands to yourself. I myself now had an illicit snack stash comprising not just juice cups and nutrition drinks, but also chips, puddings, and my new favorites, oatmeal raisin cookies. No one seemed to mind.

Then there was Tessa. No changes, for better or worse, had come to her. Always neatly dressed, her brunette curls freshly shampooed and combed, she existed in but not of the ward: unhearing, unmasked, and uncommunicative—except when complaining about a lunch thief, or when Albert chatted her up and made her smile.

By Monday evening, Sane Me and Mad Me had grown close enough to collude in a minor roast of Nurse Debra, aka the Duchess. (Well, she deserved it, after smacking me on the ass that time!) It was the own-phone hour, around eight o'clock, and I was sitting in the conference room alone, emailing friends and family with health updates. I sensed a presence in the doorway and looked up to see Nurse Annette.

"Hey, Jocelyn," she said. "Hey, um, sorry about this, but I'm going to have to ask you to move to a different room."

"A different room? Why?"

"Yeah, sorry, it's just that this room's not safe."

"Not safe?" I glanced around, confused and a little concerned. I'd been using my phone in the conference room for ten or fifteen minutes nearly every evening since I'd arrived. Now, suddenly, it wasn't safe? What was unsafe about it? The water and ice machine … the electrical outlet … the coffee swizzle sticks? "Why isn't it safe?" I asked, tensely.

Nurse Annette gave a sheepish shrug. "No, no, it's fine. It's just that Nurse Debra says it's not safe, we can't have patients in here unsupervised, and I told her look, it's Jocelyn, and I can use my judgment, but she's senior to me, so …" She shrugged again.

Aha! The picture snapped into focus. This was a room in which people—unsupervised mentally ill people, that is—would have opportunity to kill themselves. There was heavy but movable furniture. There was hot water. There were electrical cords and sharp pointy office supplies. Nurse Annette, along with Nurses Wendy, Colleen, Yvonne, et al., knew I wasn't a suicide risk and saw no reason not to let me sit in here and do email, but Nurse Annette was not in charge; Nurse Debra was, and Nurse Debra had spoken.

"Got it," I said, standing up. "No problem. Where do I go?"

"I'll put you in the staffroom, the one where you came in on your first night."

Mad Me waved a teensy red flag, and my voice went up half an octave: "Oh, OK, but you're not—you're not gonna lock the door, are you?"

"Oh, no, I won't lock the door. It's just a safer place to sit."

Don't get all stupid again, Sane Me growled. *Everything is fine.* I took my phone and followed Annette across the hall and back to that same small room with the lockers and the round table where I'd sat crying and trembling as they strip-searched me, thirteen evenings ago. It seemed remarkably nonthreatening now.

"Take your time," said Annette. She left, leaving the door ajar.

I did take my time, cognizant that Annette and I were now co-conspirators in sticking it to the Man—or rather, to Debra the Duchess. As I neared the end of my emails, Sane Me nudged me in the ribs and whispered: *You need to have some fun with this.*

Mad Me: But will the Duchess be miffed?

243

Sane Me: *So what if she is?*

Mad Me: Heh, you're right. OK, let's do it.

I walked out of the staffroom and around to the fishbowl. Nurse Annette was sitting on the other side of the sliding window doing paperwork; Nurse Debra was sitting off to the right, working on the desktop computer. I knocked on the window. When Annette opened it, I handed her my phone while saying, loud and clear:

"Please tell Debra I tried to hang myself from the doorknob, but it didn't work."

Annette cracked up, snorting into her mask. To my surprise, Debra chuckled, too. "Yeah, yeah, verrry funny," she said, fingers tapping away on the keyboard.

"Just kidding! Just kidding!" I threw the Duchess a mollifying wave and grin. Annette, still laughing, took my phone. As she slid the window shut, she winked at me.

————

A social worker, I was informed on Tuesday morning, would be coming in around eleven to square away my insurance details. At eleven a.m. precisely, the main double doors swung open and in walked ... Blonde Henchwoman! Yes, the same tall woman with short spiky hair who had trailed in the wake of the Walrus and stood, goonishly, against the wall of the intake office as I'd poured out my despair two weeks ago. Turns out she wasn't a goon at all. She introduced herself as we sat down at one of the round tables: her name was Patty, she said, and she was doing her apprenticeship in social work. "I'm new at this," (she smiled diffidently) "so please forgive me if it takes a while." It did take a while, a long while, and I had to call Matt to have him read off my insurance card numbers, which I passed along to Patty so she could enter them into the digital system, once, twice, thrice, without success, until at last she gave up and called the insurance company's 800 number. She began a long conversation with somebody while I loitered outside the fishbowl wondering if I should be helping, or at least worrying. Then the meals cart rumbled in, a pleasant glow of irresponsibility suffused me—*You've been insane, remember? No one expects YOU to help*—and I wandered off to collect my tray and eat lunch with Miranda and Reyes, leaving Patty Not-a-Goon to do battle with the bureaucracy.

Miranda was discharged that afternoon. I was engaged in a post-lunch nap on a dayroom couch as she gathered her things to head out. She had been accepted into Casa Rosa, I knew, and would be going first to the animal shelter to get her darling dog back. I was only half awake, but I heard her say, as she took her leave: "No, no, don't wake her up. Just tell her bye for me." Her voice sounded joyful. Goodbye, Gryphon, I thought; you're a good sort.

A few hours later, we had a new arrival: Michaela, a youngish woman with a husband who—judging from her side of a phone conversation with him as we both sat in the less-than-safe conference room that evening, the Duchess being off duty—was a loudmouth. Michaela had a soft round face, a soft voice, and soft brown hair, and although she talked forthrightly with her husband, it was obvious he was used to bossing his wife and was displeased about her having checked into the hospital. I wondered if she'd come to the ward partly as a way to escape his company. We had a long talk soon after her intake; she'd been placed in my room, and we sat across from each other on our twin beds, cross-legged, gabbing away like two high-school besties at a sleepover. She told me she had anxiety, which kept her from sleeping. "My family doesn't understand," she said. "My son, especially. He's seventeen. He has some mental problems. He's threatened me a few times. Physically."

"Sounds scary," I said.

"It is. I mean, it was one thing when he was little, but he's a lot bigger than me now."

"Does he live with you?"

"Yes. My husband wants to kick him out, but how can I do that? He's my son."

"Wow. I'm so sorry."

Nurse Annette walked in. "Hi, ladies! Whatcha doin?"

"We're just chatting," I said, giving her my best non-suicidal smile.

Annette smiled back, and you could see the professional wheels turning in her mind as she glanced from me, to Michaela, to me again. Apparently reassured that there were no private trachea-crushing lessons going on, she gave us an approving nod and left.

———

Wednesday, D-day, dawned clear and brisk. I got up, had breakfast, and dressed in jeans and navy-blue striped pullover. Exiting my room, I bumped into Nurse Craig, who had just arrived for the day shift.

"Morning, Jocelyn!" he said. "So, you're being discharged today. I just need to let you know, it won't be till this afternoon, because ..." His voice sank to a whisper. "Tessa is leaving this morning, and there's kind of a whole thing with that."

"Oh, sure," I said. I still felt awfully groggy in the mornings, so the point about Tessa eluded me. I just knew that today was the day, and as long as today was the day, everything was good. "Just let me know when, so I can call my husband to tell him when to pick me up. He can come any time, we live five minutes away."

Just then Nurse Yvonne came along, done with her night shift, headed for the changing room. She stopped before us and, "Look at you!" she said. "What a difference! What a *difference!*" Her accent felt like a hug. She held up her hand for a high five, and I slapped her palm, laughing. "Well done! Good luck to you!" Off she went, beaming like a proud mom.

Around nine a.m., I was ensconced on a couch at the back of the dayroom, reading My Other Book—*look, you're on page five, not bad, not bad at all*—when the two security guards showed up. They were met by Nurses Craig and Kim, and all four stood conferring for a while. I must have nodded off, for the next thing I remember is Tessa emerging from her room, Tessa in a wheelchair being pushed by Nurse Craig, a heap of luggage on her lap. Then I couldn't see what was happening, because the two guards and two nurses surrounded her, blocking my view, but after a minute the group broke up and one of the guards began pushing the wheelchair toward the back corridor, Nurse Kim and the other guard following behind. I had a clear view now.

Tessa sat passively, eyes straight ahead, right arm resting atop the bags on her lap. Her left wrist was shackled to the chair with a black handcuff and chain. She and her escorts disappeared down the hallway, and I heard a door clank open and shut. There must be a back exit, I thought. *Of course there is,* said Sane Me, *it'd be a fire hazard otherwise.* I recalled the conversation I'd had with Miranda a few days ago, when she'd filled me in on New Mexico's two major psychiatric hospitals. "The state hospital is up north, in Las Vegas," she'd said. "That one is supposed to be decent. But there's another one down south, south of Las Cruces, I forget the name. From what I hear, man, you do *not* want to be sent there."

I hope that Tessa, gentle artistic Tessa, was sent north.

———

Later that morning I attended my last Group. I don't remember what we talked about, though I remember White Queen Paula asking me how I felt about my departure, to which I replied, "It feels good, but I'm a little nervous about going home."

Paula nodded sagely. "It's perfectly normal to be a little nervous."

"Thank you, Paula. I appreciate that."

The evening before, I had spent an hour setting up a giant spiral of dominos on the long table, a hundred of them, all standing precariously on end. Paula made me promise to tell her when the display was ready for the grand knockdown. I called her over when everything was set, gave the first domino a tap, and down they went like, um, dominos: clickity-clackity-clack-clack-clack until, oh no! the third-to-last domino missed its mark, leaving the final two upright. "Aaagh!" I threw back my head and shook my fists. Nevertheless, Paula had cheered and clapped, rejoicing in my near-total success.

I'm going to miss you, White Queen, I thought as Group broke up. Not a lot, but some.

Reyes and Michaela announced they were going to do yoga and headed off to the sunroom, which had been unlocked due to the clement weather. I could hear them laughing and chatting; I was glad I was leaving Michaela with a friend. Over the past few days, I too had been upping my activity level, taking walks around and around the ward and doing occasional ballet barre exercises at the long counter under the picture windows. The vertigo had subsided to a light chop, my balance seemed better than ever, and my energy was much improved. I decided to join the two yoga-doers in the solarium.

"Hi, ladies!" I moved to one side so as not to be in their way. Thanks to the steel-mesh screens and lack of glass, the air in the sunroom was light-speckled and fresh, although the space was a bit small for three, especially since it contained a large sofa flanked by two chunky end tables. I took up a stance next to the sofa, arranged my body in the opening position for sun salutations, and proceeded to stretch my arms up and back, forward to touch my toes, one leg thrust to the rear with back arched, legs together and butt to the ceiling, stomach to the floor and arch like a cobra, fold back into child pose, then the whole thing in reverse until I was once again standing up, palms touching, elbows out. One sun salutation! Oof, I was out of breath. Reyes was doing warrior pose as Michaela splayed on the straw-matted floor in a hurdler's stretch.

"Wow, I am so out of shape," I said.

"Reyes, what's your favorite yoga pose?" asked Michaela.

"Oh, tree pose. I love tree pose." To demonstrate, Reyes stood on one leg, bent the other akimbo with the sole of that foot pressed to the opposite inner thigh, placed her palms in namaste, and held her balance admirably.

I like tree pose, too, I thought. I can do tree pose. Watch, girls, I'll show you how.

I shifted my weight to my left leg, placed my right sole on left thigh, pressed my palms together, breathed deeply like a yogi, and ... *over* to the side I went, toppling in slow motion like a felled tree. *BAM* went my left hip on the edge of the end table.

"Ow! Ow!" I staggered to my feet, pain radiating from the impact point. For a second I thought: Jesus, I've broken my hip, I am *such* an idiot. Then I thought: Well at least I won't have to go to the hospital. And then I started to laugh, because this was the first time in the whole bouncy, flouncy, trouncy trip that I'd actually lost my balance, and wouldn't losing my balance and breaking a bone on discharge day be the most marvelously ironic capstone to the whole adventure? I rubbed my hip, realized I was fine, no bones broken, and began to walk it off while Reyes and Michaela showed proper psych ward etiquette by taking no notice of the crazy lady limping around the sunroom, laughing to herself.

As for Sane Me, she took up a tree pose, balancing easily, a little smugly, somewhere above and behind my right shoulder. Had I been wearing my fleecy black hat I would have tipped it to her, but I wasn't, so I just gave her a nod and—Good job my friend, many thanks, I'll see you around. She returned the nod, her smile serene, and as she dissolved into the sempiternal sunshine of my not-so-spotless mind, I heard her say: *My work is done.*

So it came to pass that in the golden afternoon of Wednesday, November 18, 2020, I found myself exiting the St. Giles behavioral health ward through the main double doors—doors like any other doors, they were—Elephant in the crook of my arm, Nurse Craig by my side carrying the rest of my belongings in a big translucent pink garbage bag. We proceeded along the corridors, heading ever upward, it seemed to me, as if on a pilgrim's progress: no elevators to break that progress, just walking along the corridors, chatting pleasantly. My phone was sitting loose at the top of the bag; as we made a turn, it fell out onto the linoleum with a clunk. Nurse Craig said, "Oh no, your phone!" He picked it up, apologizing, and handed it to me to see if the screen had cracked. "No worries, I'm sure it's fine," I said, inwardly reveling in blithe unconcern for my stuff. I handed the phone back to him and on we walked, upward, always upward, along the corridors, with the air growing lighter, smelling fresher, until at last we came to the immense bright lobby, on the far side of which I could see the main exit, and we walked straight across the lobby and straight out the automatic doors into the boundless parking lot, with the ramp to the ER running twenty yards off to the south, the lab building hunkering a hundred yards off to the north, dozens of shiny cars waiting patiently on the asphalt, all swathed in sunlight and silence. It was the most beautiful landscape I'd ever seen.

And there was Matt, standing by the Jeep parked at the door, his eyes smiling over his facemask. I went to him, and he hugged me: "Hello, Woolly Bear!" He helped Nurse Craig put the pink garbage bag in the hatchback. I said, "Thank you" with namaste hands to Nurse Craig, who replied, "Take care, now." Then I climbed in the passenger's side, Matt got in the driver's side, and he started the engine and off we drove, gliding out of the lot, turning right and away down Hospital Drive, sailing home, home, home under a brilliant blue Santa Fe sky.

WE'RE ALL MAD HERE

As a longtime corporate-training hack, I can't resist conclud-ing with lessons learned or, as we say in the industry, take-aways. I have four.

The first, I'm sorry to say, is that when you're going insane it's advisable to have plenty of resources. Money for sure, but on top of money you'll want good insurance, a stable home life, sympathetic friends, and a supportive employer. You'll also want a healthy body, familiarity with bureaucracy, and an education that puts you at ease with complex medical information—plus the sort of demeanor, not to mention skin color, that encour-ages doctors to take you seriously and treat you with a modicum of respect. In other words: privilege. Nearly every Madlander I encountered lacked privilege, at least compared to me. Did they make it through nevertheless? I don't know. I think of them often: the Carpenter, the Fawn Girls, Savvy Alicia, Emotional Teresa ("I *feel* your dizziness!"), Kathy the Mock Turtle, Jackie the Jabberwock, Miranda the Gryphon ("That is *bull*shit!"), Coloring Girl Lindsey, Cast-foot Sam, Mad Hatter Joe ("Do ya wanna use the *phone?*") and of course, dear disconnected Tessa ("I made this for you so maybe you won't cry anymore"). I think of them all and wonder how they're doing.

Me, I'm doing well. I'm still on the Zoloft pills and the estra-diol patch, and I take progesterone and melatonin every night, 90 minutes before my boringly regular bedtime as advised by

Dr. Taylor. I weaned off the clonazepam over eighteen months, slowly and without difficulty, cutting then shaving down the pink tablets until I was taking a mouse crumb a day, then none. I still keep a small stash in case of disaster, but the bottle on the third shelf of the linen closet remains full. The mal debarquement vertigo comes and goes as feather-light turbulence, more like a raft in a pond than a boat on the ocean. The small fiber neuropathy also comes and goes, in a mildly burning band on arm, leg, or torso (it seems to have lost interest in my head), lasting a couple of weeks each time. Dr. Ortega, whom I still see semi-annually, says we'll try gabapentin if the pain gets worse. So far, it hasn't. Dr. Funar conducted her last phone appointment with me in September 2021, her Cheshire Cat smile beaming across the cellular network as she professed herself delighted with my "excellent recovery" and wished me all the best. Therapist Denise retired, leaving me without a counselor and content to keep it that way. As for sleep—beautiful bedrock sleep, never again to be taken for granted—sleep is good: when you count naps, I get a solid eight hours in each twenty-four.

Yes. I am very, very lucky.

But even if someone is not as lucky as I, there is hope. For the second big lesson I learned in Madland is that we all have a Sane Me and, when the chips are down, it's Sane Me you can count on. This guardian—whether you call her your higher self, executive function, the witness, the Word, consciousness, God, or Great Mother—is there to watch over you and *will* watch over you, stronger than the reptilian brain, more persistent than any disease, wilier than any demon. Not to say Sane Me is unvanquishable; I was separated from her, off and on, in the days leading up to my hospitalization, a state I wouldn't wish on my worst enemy. Nor would I say Sane Me alone has the power to heal; psychiatric drugs responsibly prescribed are an indispensable tool in the management of brain illnesses, as is therapy (with the caveats below). Nevertheless, if I had to point to just one guide that led me through the valley of the shadow of death, it was that bossy old bitch-angel who hovered behind my right shoulder doling out criticism, praise, and marching orders in equal portions, observing the scene with wry amusement punctuated by occasional sharp nudges in the ribs. I never heard an actual voice or felt a physical nudge. But she was real, and she is mighty.

How to nurture your Sane Me? Any serious practice will serve, I think; any discipline of body or mind that shows it's possible to feel scared, uncomfortable, sorry you signed up for this terrible gig, and to *step up anyway*. "Deep training," Matt calls it, referring to my father, who even in the depths of Alzheimer's disease retained the elegant manners required of him during his 1930s Philadelphia childhood and, later, his diplomatic career. In my case, it was ballet training that taught me I need not be controlled by the feelings of the moment, that I could (for example) hold a pose on stage for ten minutes, heart pounding, blisters burning, a dirty contact lens making one eye stream tears, then pick up my cue and go on to execute the butterfly dance to perfection. In your case, it might have been a sport, a musical instrument, the study of a science, or the practice of a faith. Anything that demands grit, for it is grit that allows our meek little oyster-self to produce pearls from suffering.

Note well, I'm not calling for the infliction of suffering as a teaching tool. Nevertheless, when human beings understand that trials in life are inevitable and, more important, that they're capable of bearing those trials with grace and courage, they do better. Everybody ought to have a good sound Sane Me, packed and ready to go, for we never know when we'll need her companionship and support.

My third takeaway is something I'd always suspected and my experiences confirmed: attributing serious mental illness to "stress" is ridiculous, and advice to "reduce stress"—whether by breathing deeply, relaxing your shoulders, talking it out, meditating, confronting your trauma, or developing coping skills—is nothing more than a convenient dictum for clinicians who don't know what's wrong with you, don't believe you when you tell them how bad it is, and don't want (or, more charitably, don't have time) to persist with the hard work of diagnosing the problem. One psychology term in particular, I think, has contributed to the lazy "it's just stress" explanation, and that term is *mood disorder*. Half a century of hearing about mood disorders has led many of us to think of mental illnesses as intensified versions of less-than-pleasant emotional states: "She's depressed" can cover anything from *She's feeling a bit sad today* all the way to *Her entire body aches, she can't tolerate light or sound, her constant thoughts are of suicide, and she hasn't been able to get out of bed for weeks.* The latter condition may look like a bad mood, but it feels like an excruciating affliction.

Mental illnesses, as I said in Chapter 7, are real illnesses. We don't put them in the same category as pneumonia or cancer, but we should. And this means that while talk therapy can no doubt help psychiatric patients cope with the emotional fallout of being brain sick (just as talk therapy can help a cancer patient cope with the emotional fallout of having cancer), I don't believe therapy has much use at all for treating the very real agony of psychiatric disease.

So what *is* useful, if not therapy?

Many people don't like to hear this, but **medications** are useful—the right ones, of course, which often take a lot of medical skill, and a lot of trial and error, to find.

Rest is useful: rest for the body, and even more for the brain. "In these cases," said Dr. Ortega, "you need to shut the brain down, just shut it down, giving it a chance to heal itself." My cure, if I boil it down to the essence, was a rest cure.

And **hospitalization** can be useful; for me, it was necessary, both to find the right meds and to permit the (moderate) shutdown that allowed my brain to rest and heal.

"But," you ask, "can't people do that on an outpatient basis?" Maybe some can. I couldn't. If I had it to do over, I'd go to the hospital a lot sooner. I'd travel through looking-glass world much faster, jumping from square to chessboard square, jousting with Red Queens and White Queens until they crowned me Queen of the Remote and set me free. I'd ask for—no, *demand*—medical help much earlier. I would understand that, for most of us, Madland is the way through and out of hell, not the way in.

Which leads me to the final takeaway.

Mental illness is another country, a country full of curious, fabulous, thoroughly human monsters. Like Alice, I did not want to go among them, yet, "We're all mad here" said the Cat, and an insanity excursion might be one we all must make at some point in our travels through this vast, baffling universe, lest we persist in the arrogant belief that *we* could never go zipping off to the Bad Place on a ticket we don't remember having bought, that *we* could never be guest of honor at a Mad Tea Party. In truth, any of us may suddenly and inexplicably find ourselves running as fast as we can just to keep in one spot, with the earth churning beneath our feet, a superior Caterpillar shouting "green, Denver, horse!" and a jovial Vaseline Man jogging alongside. Anyone might slip through the looking glass or down the rabbit hole. Anyone can take a wild ride to Madland.

I certainly don't recommend it as something to do, but I'll say this:

It is something to have done.

THE END

ACKNOWLEDGMENTS

The day I got out of the hospital, Matt made dinner for us; Trader Joe's meatloaf, I think it was, with peas on the side and milk to drink. Before picking up my beautifully pointy, non-plastic fork, I proposed a toast: "To modern medicine!"

"How strange," you say, "that after such a horrible medical ordeal with so much ineffective medical advice, you'd want to make *that* toast."

Maybe it was strange, but as I wrote in the Prologue:

> When I look back at my time in Madland, I see
> ... some violently damaged souls and a few coldly
> calloused ones; mostly, though, I see a lot of caring,
> competent medical pros going to work every day and
> trying their best, within the limits of a flawed system,
> to treat a lot of perfectly ordinary, unaccountably
> screwed-up patients who persist bravely in seeking
> treatment for their ill-understood conditions.

The way I see it, 80 percent of the credit for my recovery, hence for this book, goes to those workaday medical pros. In particular, and still without giving their real names, I want to thank:

- Dr. Ortega, my stalwart primary care physician
- Dr. Cook, the Knave of Hearts who taught me all about vertigo
- Dr. Funar, my insightful and generous psychiatrist with the Cheshire Cat smile

- the attending doctors of the St. Giles Behavioral Health Ward
- White Queen Paula, kind counselor and Group leader
- the Mayo Clinic Scottsdale Neurology department, especially Smart Nurse and Dr. "You Just Got in a Funk" Goodman

But above all, I want to thank Nurses Wendy, Annette, Craig, Kim, Yvonne, Priya, Colleen, Debra, and the rest. I trust they will recognize themselves despite the pseudonyms. When fighting demons, you need angels on your side; those psych ward nurses were, and still are, my angels.

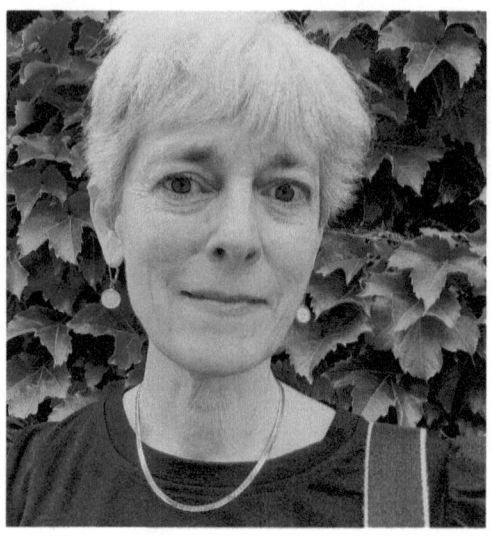

Jocelyn Davis is a retired consulting executive turned author with master's degrees in philosophy and Eastern classics. Her previous leadership books include *Strategic Speed, The Greats on Leadership, The Art of Quiet Influence,* and *Insubordinate.* Her historical novel, *The Age of Kali,* has been called "brilliant," "heretical," and "deeply moving." Jocelyn grew up in a foreign-service family, living in Southeast Asia, East Africa, and the Caribbean. Currently she lives in Santa Fe, New Mexico, with her husband, Matt, and a small community of senior stuffed animals of which Elephant is queen.

Visit her website at JocelynRDavis.com.

www.ingramcontent.com/pod-product-compliance
Lightning Source LLC
Chambersburg PA
CBHW030411130626
46549CB00004B/1727